# HerbsRx

*Traditional and indigenous alternatives to conventional medications*

*Alkaline, Traditional Chinese Medicine, Ayurveda and natural herbs used to treat Disease*

**STEFAN WOMACK**

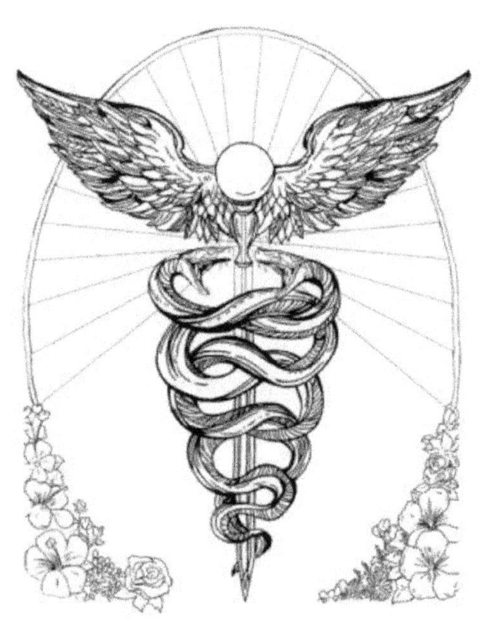

# Table of Contents

# Introduction

My journey into the world of pharmaceutical was one driven by my love of science. While taking classes in college, I decided that I wanted to pursue a career to become a pharmacist. One piece of advice that I got was to work in a pharmacy to see if you would enjoy that employment. So with no prior knowledge of medicine, I applied to become a pharmacist technician. I figured out the best way to learn about a subject is to work in that field. I wound up getting the job that would alter my life and give me knowledge and insight into the world of medicine. After getting hired I was literally reading every book and piece of information I could to learn about different medicine names, brand or generic, which medicine was used for what and so forth. While working I was still taking all the science classes required for applying to pharmacy school. After a couple of years going into my employment, I started to notice some interesting insights into the world of medicine. There were a lot of different medications that treated the same disease. Next, the amount of money that is made and generated from a customer is insane. I've personally seen people on the same medications for 10+ years and they are just maintaining, but never really healing. Therein lies the trap. If someone can keep you at a certain level, but not heal you they have a customer for life. Money cannot be made if a disease is cured, profit can only be made if that disease is only "treated". A year into my path I became certified and registered with the board of pharmacy as a technician. While working in the pharmacy my love for science never stopped I was constantly reading all the prescription label information from all the manufactures. Most people would throw those in the trash but I would take these home and study these to learn about the chemistry of what was being dispensed to people. During this time I also found my true calling which was the study and uses of herbs and fruits as medicine. Also called alternative medicine. This was really fascinating to me because this was a complete opposite of what I was doing for a living. Years and years down the line of studying all different cultures and philosophies I came to realize that the non-conventional way of healing was far superior to the conventional way of treating disease. About 2 years ago I got the opportunity to become a health presenter with The City of Atlanta. This gave me the chance to impart some of my acquired knowledge with my class. My class was mostly seniors. They were the most rewarding students I have ever encountered. Never in my wildest dreams did I think I would be getting paid to speak on health. One of the most rewarding experiences was hearing about people who were able to "cure" some previous 'incurable" disease. Hearing those stories let me know I was on the right path. One of the main reasons I gravitated towards the non-conventional approach was because of a simple physical law that cannot be broken. If everything was created perfect and in harmony with nature and its naturally at a ratio of 100%, how can man create something from a product that will ever be in accordance with nature or even be able to be at 100% effectiveness Almost all if not all prescription drugs come from something that was isolated from something in nature or created in a lab. A perfect example would be acetaminophen (Tylenol, Aspirin). The ancient people of Kemet (Egypt) used willow bark as a remedy for aches and pains as far back as 6000 years ago. One of the components of willow bark is salicylic acid, which reduces body temperature and helped decrease inflammation in the body. Hippocrates, the Greek physician who learned and stole everything from his teachers in Kemet (Egypt) also wrote that willow bark and leaves also had the same effects. But a boundary is crossed when Man takes from Nature (God) and tries to capitalize on its components. In the 1800's salicylic acid was finally isolated from the willow bark. When you isolate a particular compound that's when it becomes a DRUG! So what's wrong with that you may ask? What other medicinal properties did the whole willow bark have? What process was done chemically to isolate the desired compound? How does the body react to the isolated compound and not the whole plant? Is the isolated compound alkaline or acidic? These are questions that western medicine tends to negate. Now I have to be clear there is definitely a need for highly skilled surgeons and people in emergency situations. The problem lies in the general practice of the common physician. Question, why do pharmaceutical companies have sell reps. These "drug" reps go from doctor office to doctor office and pharmacy to pharmacy providing "gifts" and incentives for them to dispense their products. According to public records in 2016 alone over 6 billion dollars were paid by drug companies to doctors (those are just the disclosed payments). Over 800,000 doctors and over 1,700 hospitals received payments. Source (https://projects.propublica.org). Not only do they get paid to see and "treat" you, they get paid to prescribe certain medications that profit them. Now ask yourself do they really care about you or do they care about their own income. The blame doesn't lie in the pharmacist or the doctor, it lies in the system which teaches and governs them. The traditional system has many flaws in it. The main flaw is an overlook of basic chemistry, biological, and physics of the body. The drive to create different products that generate more income for a pharmaceutical company, leads man more and more from an Organic approach to a more Inorganic approach. I've been working in the pharmaceutical field for more than 8 years. At any given time there is more than 500 different medications in stock and 1000s more available thru online ordering. The further you get from nature the closer you get to the grave! Nothing created from a plant, herb, or fruit will be better than the actual thing. It will never happen. It's so simple yet so complicated to understand this concept. Nature has a cure for every Dis-ease, man has a treatment for every Dis-ease. That's why it's called a treatment center, can't cure but can just treat and suppress the symptoms but not the actual root cause with synthetics. One of the biggest factors I have seen is a disease of the mind. The average person is so laxed and comfortable that they hardly question anything anymore. I always told my seniors to question everything, included the information I was presenting. Nobody will ever have your greater interest in mind other than yourself. You are your own healer

# Chapter 1: Basic and Fundamental Chemistry

What is the human body? The body is made of up roughly 37 trillion cells as well as over 100 trillion bacteria! That means from the top of our heads to the bottom of our feet we are literally nothing but chemical reactions taking place. The body is made up of up between 50% to 75% water. Majority of the water in the body is contained in our cells. Understanding this is crucial for every human being. Every organ in our bodies is nothing but a collection of cells that are serving a particular function that comes together perfectly like a gigantic jigsaw puzzle. If you're looking at the heart, hair, liver, or prostate it's all just a bunch of cells. Nature doesn't do randomness, everything is always done with a Divine intelligence that man will never truly grasp. Just like every other organism on this earth, cells eat for energy and expel waste. Waste is a byproduct of a chemical reaction, IE (industrial waste, biological waste, atmospheric waste). This is the reason people eat, they have to feed trillions and trillions of cells from the day they are born unto death. The main reason so much disease is present is the body's inability to get rid of all the cellular wastes. Disease is literally broken down to Dis (meaning lack of) and Ease (meaning physical comfort, undisturbed state of the body). Disease is a lack of something physical not moving in the body. We all know the answer to what that physical something is, its Waste!!! On average from the mouth to the anus is a distance of 30 feet. That's how far our food has to travel in the body to get properly digested. It takes 6 to 8 hours just to reach the small intestines alone. For full digestion, it ranges from 12 to 16 hours. The thing about Americans is the consistency and over indulgence of food. If you eat 3 meals a day plus 2 snacks for 60 years just imagine how much waste is built up and stored in the body. Simple math, let's say it takes 12 hours to fully digest your first meal completely. You then eat 3 meals a day and no snacks, that's 12*3= 36. There are only 24 hours in a day, so in theory, it would take you at least 1.5 days to digest 3 meals from the previous day with no food on that day. Now we can see where the buildup of waste over time happens. If this same person continued the same pattern for 60 years, disease and other ailments would be a guaranteed. On average the human body from mouth to anus is connected by a 30 feet or 9-meter tube. To put that in comparison that's the length of 4 Shaquille O' Neil (7'1 ft) standing on top of each other! That's a long way to travel after each meal. That's why people get sluggish and tired after eating a big unhealthy meal. The body has to do a lot of work to process all that has been ingested. In Physics, the definition of Work is the measure of energy transfer that happens when an object is displaced over a distance by an external force at least some of which is applied in the direction of the initial displacement. By that definition alone every time we eat we should be mindful of how much work we are causing our body to perform.

# Minerals of the body

One of my favorite Quotes of all time came from Linus Pauling. Who is Linus Pauling you may ask? He was one of four people in History to receive two Nobel Prizes in the field of Science. He stated that "you can trace every sickness, every disease and every ailment to a mineral deficiency". Just that Quote alone should tell you how important minerals are to the body. A look at the study of medicine from the western approach is as follows: Genes are at the top, then neurotransmitters, also hormones, followed by enzymes and lastly is Vitamins. The problem is that minerals are never talked about. Vitamins won't work in the body if there aren't any minerals present. That's like a car running with no source of energy to propel it. Minerals must be available for vitamins to work. Once that Vitamin does its work, it's called a co-enzyme. An enzyme is a vitamin, amino acid, and a mineral working together to make something happen. No minerals mean no vitamins that do work and become enzymes. Hormones and neurotransmitters are produced by enzymes. No minerals, subsequently mean no vitamins that turn to enzymes that produce hormones and neurotransmitters. And lastly genes, which are bathed in vitamins, minerals and enzymes from the day you are born till the day you die. Minerals are the Architect and foundation of every metabolic process in the body. Thus the importance of understanding how and which minerals our body needs to operate and maintain homeostasis.

Let's look at the ratio between minerals of the human body and the Earth's crust:

| Elements | Human Body | Earth's Crust |
|---|---|---|
| Oxygen | 65% | 49% |
| Carbon | 18% | <1% |
| Hydrogen | 10% | <1% |
| Nitrogen | 3% | trace |
| Calcium | 2% | 3% |
| Iron | <0.05% | 5% |
| Aluminum | <0.001% | 8% |
| Silicon | Trace | 26% |

One thing to take Note in the above chart is the ratio of the human body that is made up of Oxygen, Carbon, and

Hydrogen. 93% that's literally almost the whole body Cells run on Carbon (which is sugar) and Oxygen. Carbon is like the gas for your cells and gives them the fuel to burn. Oxygen is like the spark for the gas to be ignited. If you don't get sugars (fructose, glucose, or galactose) your cells will not eat and function properly. Fructose, glucose and galactose are broken down into Carbon, which is the bases to Carbohydrates, which are carbon chain substituents. There are simple, poly, and complex carbohydrates. Simple carbohydrates are all fruits and some vegetables. Poly and complex are called starch. Human beings run exclusively on these constituents, especially simple carbohydrates. All organic chemistry is based on the study of carbon and carbon chains. We are Carbon based beings. We take in oxygen from the air and mix with carbon at the cellular level to get ATP (adenosine- triphosphate), which is basically the energy for all of the cells. Here is a look at some other key minerals in the body and their functions.

- Chromium- sugar metabolism and mineral cofactor

- Phosphorous- tooth and muscle formation

- Calcium- tooth and muscle formation, cardiovascular health, strong bones and teeth

- Manganese- bone health
- Zinc- brain, cellular and immune functions
- Potassium- blood pressure, sends oxygen to the brain
- Copper- metabolic process
- Magnesium- heart regulation, relaxes muscles
- Selenium- immune function
- Chlorine- aids in digestion (hydrochloric acid)
- Silicon- bone and connective tissue health
- Sulfur-healthy hair, skin, and nails
- Sodium- nerve and muscle function
- Iodine-thyroid function

# Acid and Base (Alkaline)

Our bodies prefer to be in an alkaline environment. The pH of the blood of human beings is slightly alkaline normally in the range of 7.35 to 7.45. Why is this important to note?? Let's explain a little general chemistry. In chemistry, we have reactions that occur on every level. Most if not all reactions are done in a solution, in our case the liquid in our bodies. When a chemical reaction takes place something is either gained or lost. Since water ($H_2O$) is the most common solution found on earth and in our body we test for the lost or gain of Hydrogen (H) atoms by a pH test. That test ranges from 0 to 14. Water being the medium its pH is 7. Anything below 7 is considered from slightly acidic to very acid. Anything above 7 is considered to be slightly basic to a strong base. All of our 37 trillion cells and 100 trillion bacteria are surrounded by fluids in our body. These fluids are called interstitial fluids. The most known is, of course, blood plasma, which stated is slightly alkaline. The other is tissue fluid and lymph fluid. Blood Plasma in the blood contains water, proteins, nutrients, ions, hormones and some waste. Tissue Fluid bathes the tissues; similar to blood plasma but has no proteins. Lymph is tissue fluid that is drained into the lymphatic system. So, in essence, in essence every chemical reaction between our cells is surrounded these fluids that govern and regulate every aspect of biological function for a human being. All these reactions taking place tend to find favor in a slightly alkaline solution.

Acidity and Alkalinity and the balance between those two is the bases of health. But this also correlates with the old saying As Above So Below. We live in a world of masculine and feminine energy. There is a fine line between the balance of those two but we all must walk the line and find Peace, which is, in essence, in essence finding homeostasis. Acid is the masculine side of chemistry. An acid in science gives up its Hydrogen proton willingly, it's called a proton donor. Acids are volatile and corrosive. They are essential but too much can very detrimental. Just like a boy likes to break something down to see its components and try to understand the structure. Like a toy, car, computer etc. the masculine energy is associated with the left side of the brain. The left side performs duties such as logic and reasoning. Like mathematics, architecture and science. The right side of the brain is the feminine side, it's alkaline based. The right side of the brain is linked to creativity and arts. Like music, drawing, love and compassion. A base in science is classified as a proton acceptor. That means a base accepts the Hydrogen given off from the Acid in a chemical reaction. In our body for instance in the stomach is found Hydrochloric acid which has a pH of 1 to 3, which on the pH scale is extremely acidic. But it's needed to break down the waste and bacteria in the human body. On the other hand, the Pancreas gland, which is part of the lymph system produces sodium bicarbonate in the body to counter too much acid and ranges from 7 to 8.2 pH. Normal skin pH is around 5.5 making it acidic. The body always finds a way to find peace, homeostasis. The saliva in our mouth and throughout the body is 7.1 to 7.5 pH on a healthy person, making it slightly alkaline. Meaning that whenever we put something too acidic in the body that wasn't made from nature a WAR starts. Chemistry governs every function of this existence. The further we go back in time we find that we were mainly alkaline based. We ate berries, fruits and some vegetables for the most part before our diets were changed to ACID base. The bases of an Acid based diet is pain and inflammation. Too much unnatural acids in the body is a direct correlation to the intake of high Acidic foods and inflammation. What is considered an Acid forming food? All animal products, animal by-products, most grains, most legumes, and even some nuts. You can now start to see a trend starting to form with what the body is made of and needs and the difference between what your taste buds want. We have to learn how to eat for nutrition and not for taste. The average American taste buds are so conditioned for Acidic foods from years and years of constant bombardment of manmade junk, refined carbohydrates, and tons and tons of animal flesh. Just something to think about the average pH of soft drinks is 2 to 2.5. That's extremely acidic but kids start drinking this at a younger and younger age with no flinch. That's scary the taste buds have been fried to the point that they actually crave something that can peel paint! Acidosis is a condition caused by an overproduction of acid in the blood plasma or an excessive loss of sodium bicarbonate from the blood called metabolic acidosis, or by an accumulation of carbon dioxide in the blood that results from poor lung function or decreased breathing called respiratory acidosis. If an increase in acid comes into the body and affects the body's acid-base homeostasis. A signal in the brain goes off that regulates breathing are stimulated to produce faster and deeper breathing (respiratory compensation). The kidneys try and compensate by putting out more acid in the urine. But conversely, the body can become too overwhelmed if the body continues to produce too much acid, leading to severe Acidosis and eventually to heart problems and coma. Acidosis has 2 pathways into the body Metabolic and Respiratory. In metabolic acidosis, it occurs when the amount of acid in the body is raised from consuming substances that are broken down to (metabolized) to an acid. Also, a malfunctioning metabolism can produce metabolic acidosis. Even the production of normal amounts of acid can lead to acidosis when the kidneys aren't functioning optimally and cannot excrete enough amounts of acid in the urine. Respiratory acidosis occurs when the lungs can't expel carbon dioxide sufficiently, a problem that can arise that affect the lungs like pneumonia, bronchitis, and asthma. Respiratory acidosis can also arise when brain malfunctions or the nerves and muscles of the chest impair breathing. Another pathway for respiratory acidosis comes when the breathing slows down in the body from the over intake of opioids (narcotics) or strong prescription drugs for sleep (sedatives). One question I have is the prescription drug your taking hurting or helping you. Is it acidic or alkaline? If it doesn't come from the earth 9 times out 10 it's acidic. If your medication is acidic it steals minerals from you. Making your body work twice as hard to fight the disease and the loss of minerals from the drugs. One last thing on pH before we move on. You cannot change the pH of your blood, if that happens you would die instantly. On contrary, your other fluids in your body can be affected by the rise and fall of your pH levels. That's why it's best to ultimately transition to a plant-based diet. If it came from an animal it's acidic, there are no beneficial animal products, none!

# **Electricity**

A battery is, in essence, a representation of the human body. A battery works on the principle of two different minerals separated by a salt bridge that allows the flow of positive and negative electrons to create power. Our body runs on electricity, the brain and the nervous system are electrical. The brain communicates thru synapsis which is identical to an electrical charge in a battery. The better the flow of electricity in the body, the stronger and faster the brain and nervous system can respond. It's essential to eat foods that are highly electrical. What are electrical foods? Foods that contain minerals of course, real, organic, preferably uncooked fruits and vegetables. The more food a person eats that is not mineral-rich the more electricity is lost and is affected. Just like a battery eventually runs out of power, so will the body. The nervous system runs thru out the entire body. Every reflex, breath, action, and thought requires electricity for that to happen. The nervous system is like the blood veins for an electrical current. Carrying the pulse to the desired parts of the body almost instantly. If you want to test the speed of your electrical current stub your toe on a bedpost. You will quickly see and feel the speed of the nervous system!! In the human body, there are often pairs of minerals that have to be in a certain ratio like in a battery to function properly. Sodium (Na) and Potassium (K) which should be at a 1 to 5 ratio to maintain optimal health, but in America its 2 to 1, that means most people have too much sodium in their diet. Another one is Cooper (Cu) to Zinc (Zn) which should be at (8 to 1) to (12 to 1) ratio for perfect health. Copper and Zinc work synergistically to promote immune response, nervous system functions, and digestion. Copper and Zinc are antagonistic in relation, meaning if one is out of balance the other will rise. Some common occurrences of excess copper and deficient zinc can lead to headaches, anxiety, hair loss, depression and impaired memory just to name a few. Calcium (Ca) and Magnesium (Mg) in America it's a 4 to1 ratio between (Ca) vs (Mg), but it should be at a 1 to 1 ratio (Ca) to (Mg). Calcium and Magnesium also have a synergistic relationship. If one is out of hand the other will suffer. Americans take in the most amount of Calcium in the world, but still, have the highest rate of osteoporosis. Magnesium is needed for the synthesis of Vitamin D in the body. Vitamin D is used to fortify the bones and make them stronger. In essence, a lack of magnesium and too much calcium is properly related to the brittle bones epidemic in this country. The older a person gets they are more prone to experience mental fatigue and exhaustion, could that be related to a slowing down of the electrical connections in the brain. We lose minerals on daily bases thru sweat, using the restroom, or being filtered thru our kidneys. It's quite important every day to replenish those minerals lost so you can keep the electricity flowing!

# Chapter 2: Alkaline/Electric, TCM, and Auryvedic Principles

Dr. Sebi was a great inspiration to myself and countless others. I never got a chance to personally meet him or have I ever been to Usha Village in Honduras. Fortunately, I was able to come across Dr. Sebi thru YouTube. When I heard his philosophy on health and nutrition as well as his life story I was instantly drawn to him. I was up all night watching video after video. Learning and listening to the master teacher/ healer. If it wasn't for his teachings I would of never loss over 100 lbs and transform my life forever. In one of his early video's Dr. Sebi said when he was younger he read a book by Arnold Ehret that changed his life. Arnold Ehret claim to fame was the mucusless diet. Healing the body thru fasting and getting rid of excess mucus in the body. His philosophy, as well as a majority of Dr. Sebi was as follows. First, a 2 to 3-day detox was always recommended. If the body has excess mucus and waste you want to help get the waste moving. It's always best to do a detox at least 4 times a year. Secondly, fasting was the key to health, doing extensive fasts periodically was beneficial for the body. Allowing the body to selfheal was a priority. Also, when breaking fast the best choice is always fruits, usually because of the high water content and fiber. They both advocated a plant based lifestyle as the optimum diet for people to eat. One difference was that Dr. Sebi taught about herbs and how useful and helpful they can be if applied to daily use. Dr. Sebi used his knowledge of herbs to create plenty of herbs and tonics to help heal the body. Many celebrities sought out his service before his untimely Death in 2016.

Traditional Chinese Medication (TCM) may be the second oldest practice outside of Africa to have such an extensive history of Herbs and healing. According to Orient lore, Li Ch'ing Yuen was said to have lived for over 250 years of age before his death. Chinese modern scholars have verified his lifespan. Born in 1678 and deceased in 1930. It is said he used TCM every day throughout his life and also practiced yoga. There are so much different topics to cover the whole aspect of TCM in one section. So here is a brief overview of this philosophy. Everything is energy. Nothing is separate from the whole. Man is a conduit between the earth and the heavens. Both transmitting and receiving energy from both. In TCM Ch'i is the word for energy. Food is energy, air is energy, and thoughts are energy. Even in the body, there are energy meridian channels. They call the opposite flow of energy Yin and Yang. According to Taoist master Huang-Keu "the yin conserves and the yang radiates". One example would be the Autonomic Nervous System, which has 2 components called the parasympathetic and sympathetic. The parasympathetic component is primarily directed towards the preservation, reserve, and housing of energies in the body. On the contrary, the effect of the sympathetic nervous stem is antagonistic because it causes the output of bodily energies and blocks the absorption of nutrient matter. The human body functions under the dual control of the autonomic nervous system. The body is filled with Ch'i and it radiates to our aura. Not until recently this was a speculated subject, but with the invention of Kirlian photography which has confirmed the existence of an aura field around all living objects. Research into the old saying a "green thumb" is really true. It has been proven that a person can radiate energy which is beneficial to a plants aura. Vice versa a person with a "brown thumb" does the opposite with their energy emitted. In TCM there are

| traditionally 5 primary flavors: | Which also affect major organs in the body: |
| --- | --- |
| Wood = sour flavor | Wood Ch'i effects Liver and Gall Bladder |
| Fire =bitter flavor | Fire Ch'i effects Heart, Small Intestines, Circulation-Sex |
| Earth =sweet flavor | Earth Ch'i effects Spleen-Pancreas and Stomach |
| Metal =pungent (or spicy) flavor | Metal Ch'i effects Lung and Large Intestine |
| Water =salty flavor | Water Ch'i effects Kidney and the Bladder |

In TCM the Ch'i located in the body provides energy to 12 different meridians in the body that herbs are said to effect. The system is broken into six pairs, one with a Yin quality the other a Yang Quality. Each has an elemental quality as well.

1) The Lungs – Yin organ system affected by Metal Ch'i. The lungs regulate the Ch'i, skin, pores, larynx, sinuses and diaphragm.

2) The Large Intestines – Yang counterpart to the lungs affected by Metal Ch'i. The large intestine is used to transporting solid waste from the body. Also, effects the water levels in the body and the purity of bodily fluids.

3) The Stomach – Yang organ and affected by Earth Ch'i. In TCM Ch'i is extracted from food in the stomach. Often called the "Sea of Nourishment", used for nutrient extraction for the body. Also said to affect metabolism.

4) The Spleen – Yin organ and affected by Earth Ch'i. Influences the function of the pancreas. The spleen helps influence fluid circulation and distribution and works with the Kidneys in regulating the amount of fluid kept in the body. Helps refine and regulate the quality of the blood.

5) The Heart- Yin organ affected by Fire Ch'i. Unlike western thought in TCM, the heart controls the functions of the cerebral cortex and the limbic center of the brain that controls our emotions. Rules the cardiovascular system and the transport of blood thru out the body. The heart function includes the thyroid and thymus gland as well.

6) The small intestines- Yang organ affected by Fire Ch'i. Used for the separation of food into its organic and inorganic components. The site where bacteria activity is crucial for essential nutrient absorption. Connected

to the pituitary gland, which produces crucial hormones that are necessary for nearly all aspects of organic life, and is called the master gland.

7) The Bladder – Yang organ affected by Water Ch'i. Regulates the gathering and expel of urine. Helps balance the parasympathetic and sympathetic nervous system in the body.

8) The Kidney – Yin organ affected by Water Ch'i. The kidney in TCM considered the "Root of Life". Filters the blood, removes cellular waste and excess water as well. The kidneys regulate the acid/base relationship of bodily fluids in the body through series of reactions involving minerals like potassium, sodium, ammonia, and bicarbonate. The kidneys include the adrenal glands as well, which control the production of hormones and steroids in the body. Also, the kidneys are associated with controlling the hair on the head, facial hair and pubic hair.

9) The Gall Bladder- Yang organ affected by Wood Ch'i. Regulates the flow of bile in the body, which is needed for digestion of fat and oily foods.

10) Circulation-Sex- Usually associated with the pericardium, the heart's protective casing a Yin fire system. In western term, it is similar to the spirit. Influences the feeling of love that is expressed sexually as a link between emotion and sexual intercourse.

11) The Triple Warmer- Yang and Fire, associated with the hypothalamus, a part of the brain responsible for many everyday bodily functions like producing Hormones, appetite, body temperature regulation and many more.

12) The Liver- Yin organ affected by Wood ch'i. The liver is where the blood in the body flows to get detoxified. The liver houses a large portion of sugar in the form of Glycogen, which is available to go into the bloodstream when needed for work. All the proteins and hormones in the body are broken down in the liver. The peripheral nervous system (nerves stemming from the central nervous system) is connected to the liver in TCM, which has a direct link to the eyes and vision of the body as well. In the act of sexual intercourse, the Liver is said to provide energy to the sex organs.

Ayurveda dates back at least 7000 years and was cultivated by Indians and Hindus. Ayurveda has different branches of study. One branch of study is Rasayana. Ras= primordial tissue or plasma and ayana= path. The origin of the word means the path of plasma. In the different branches of study, Rasayana is the field associated with body rejuvenation. In Ayurveda, the lifespan of the human is broken down into 4 different stages.

1) From birth to about 20 years old, all bodily tissues are growing

2) 20 to 40 years old, tissues still growing

3) 40 to 60 the age of plateau. Alternatively, if a person has a good diet, great mindset, free of worry and anxiety, this stage can be used to expand mental fortitude.

4) From 60 on, no matter a high quality of life, certain functions slow down. Like metabolism, bone and tendon loss as well as mental cognition decrease.

For stages 3 and 4 that's where Rasayana was especially useful for rejuvenation of the body. Similar to TCM, the study of Rasayana is to correct the balance of the body by different ras (associated with a different taste). Whatever goes into our mouth has one or more of 6 ras.

1) Sweet ras- mainly found in carbohydrates like starch and sugar-containing products, fuels bones, semen, blood, liver and flesh. In overabundance causes laziness, diabetes, high blood pressure, as well as obesity.

2) Acidic ras- commonly associated with acidic fruit and fermented food. Affects saliva, increases digestion. In access can acidify the body.

3) Salty ras- found in minerals, makes food palatable. Excess of salt can increase thirst, hair loss and a loss of sexual vigor.

4) Bitter ras- main constitute of herbs. Alkalize the body, removes cellular waste, and strengths and fortifies the body. In excess can be an anti-inflammatory catalyst.

5) Pungent ras- Spices, used to give food zest and flavor. Help get rid of microbes in the food. Excess can initiate sedation and laziness.

6) Astringent ras- generally in unripe fruit, barks and roots. In excess can cause detriment to the nervous system.

As well as the 6 ras there are 3 different doshas. Vata, Pitta, and Kapha, these are equivalent to air, bile, and phlegm. They have a synergy with the different ras and are affected differently by each. Sweet ras decreases vata, sweet and pungent ras decreases pitta and so forth.

Vata is the life force of the body associated with air. It separates cells into other structures, creates blood vessels and nerves. If vata remains in order all five senses will remain stable, if not disease or death could occur.

Pitta produces and maintains body heat associated with bile. Used in digestion, metabolic activity and nutrient assimilation. Closely associated with the liver and spleen to generate blood. Too much spicy, fried sour and salty food can cause an excess of pitta. Excess pitta can lead to a loss of calcium, acidity or headaches.

Kapha associated with phlegm has a cooling aspect and provides the right condition for bile, mucous membranes and gastric juices. Kapha is affected by sweet, sour and hard to digest foods. Causes the common cold, cough, and bronchial flare-ups. Increases mucus and saliva production.

# Chapter 3: The Profit of Disease

The number of people who took at least one prescription drug in the last 30 days including both men and women and all races. 1988-1994 =39.1%, 1999-2002=45.2%, 2007-2010=47.5% and 2011-2014= 47.0%

The number of people on three or more prescription drugs in the last 30 days including both sexes and races. 1988-1994=11.8%, 1999-2002=17.8%, 2007-2010=20.8% and 2011-2014=21.5%

The number of people on five or more prescription drugs in the past 30 days including both sexes and races. 1988-1994=4.0%, 1999-2002=7.5%, 2007-2010=10.1% and 2011-2014=10.9%

As you can see the number has been on a constant increase for almost 20 years. It's been estimated that at least 70 % of the American population is taking at least one prescription drug on the regular.

**Here is a list of Pharmaceutical Company's revenue in 2015 and 2016**

1) Johnson and Johnson; 70.04 billion and 71.89 billion

2) Pfizer; 48.85 billion and 52.82 billion

3) Roche; 47.70 billion and 50.11 billion

4) Novartis; 49.41 billion and 48.52 billion

5) Merck; 29.5 billion and 39.8 billion

6) Sanofi; 36.73 billion and 36.57 billion

7) GlaxoSmithKline; 29.84 billion and 34.79 billion

8) Gilead Sciences; 32.15 billion and 30.39 billion

9) AbbVie; 22.82 billion and 25.56 billion

10) Bayer; 24.09 billion and 25.27 billion

Just those 10 companies alone profited over 300 billion dollars alone each year. Now you can see the money behind Big Pharmaceutical. Drug companies have drug reps who go from physician office to physician office pushing their employer's product. Drug reps even come to the pharmacy to push their products. Did you know Doctor's get incentives from pharmaceutical companies for dispensing a particular drug over another, not because one is better but because the doctor will get a kickback the more patients are on that particular medication? Under President Obama healthcare law, drug companies are required to make public their payouts to Doctors. Analyst uses the law and created the tool Open Payments, where patients can see if a conflict of interest exists when prescribed a certain prescription or medical device. One pharmaceutical company in 2015 spent over $36,000,000 in general payments and $45,000,000 in research payments alone. While saying "Compensation for services other than consulting, including serving at faculty or as a speaker at a venue other than a continuing education program". That same pharmaceutical company the same year paid 2 physicians over $600,000 for prescribing certain prescriptions. This is not to say Doctors are all out to make extra money. The fact is the Big drug companies have essentially bout out the medical field. It has been estimated going back 20 years at least 100,000 people die annually from adverse reactions from prescription medications. An article in the 1998 American Medical Association projected 106,000 deaths that year alone. As far as recent projections the number is over 125,000 deaths annually. Professor Donald Light at the Rowan University of Osteopathic Medicine says "about 2,460 people per week are estimated to die from drugs that were properly prescribed, and that's based on detail chart reviews of hospitalized patients".

The Number needed to treat and the Number needed to harm are two key concepts that most people haven't heard of before. Every prescription drug that reaches the market has to be tested for its safety and effectiveness. After the testing is done and the results come back a Number needed to treat is given. This means that for every 1 person that benefits from that drug a certain number of people either experience no effect or a side effect from that drug. An example would be low dose Aspirin (acetaminophen), said to help lower the risk of a heart attack. Let's look at the Number needed to treat, 1 in 1667 for one year. That means that for every 1667 people taking low dose aspirin daily for 1 year, only 1 person will prevent a cardiovascular problem. The number needed to treat for a person to prevent a non-life threatening heart attack is 1 in 2000 for one year. For the prevention of Strokes, low dose Aspirin is also recommended to take. The number needed to treat is 1 in 3000 for one year. For every 3000 people taking this medication only 1 person will prevent a non-life threatening stroke.

The number needed to harm is the inverse of the number needed to treat. It calculates the average number of people, taking a certain prescription over time to be exposed to a negative effect that caused harm against one person who would not be affected. Staying with low dose Aspirin the number needed to harm is 1 in 3333 for one year. For every 3333 people taking low dose aspirin daily for one year, 1 person was "harmed", which in the case of low dose aspirin was a major bleeding incident.

# Chapter 4. Thyroid

Thyroid medication is one of the most prescribed drugs in America. It's consistently in the top 3 prescribed drugs annually. A lot of people have thyroid conditions, some even have to have the thyroid gland removed through surgery. What exactly are the thyroid gland and its role in the body? The thyroid gland is part of the endocrine system of the human body. The endocrine system is similar to the nervous system, these 2 are the master systems of the body. They regulate and govern the other body systems. The endocrine system produces and delivers chemical messengers called hormones throughout the body. Hormones are like an on and off switch in the cells, it tells the cells to do a certain job function or stop doing a certain job function. There are glands that have different functions in the body like the thalamus gland, pituitary gland, adrenal glands, pineal gland, ovaries and testes, which all produce various hormones. Located in the neck just in front of the larynx, the thyroid gland produces two main hormones thyroxine and triiodothyronine. Thyroxine main function is to initiate consumption of Oxygen thus fueling metabolism of all cells and tissues in the body.

Thyroxine is referred to as T4 and triiodothyronine is referred to as T3. Thyroxine (T4) is the messenger hormone of the thyroid gland, it gets produced in the thyroid gland and flows in the bloodstream to its desired cells where it's converted to T3. When converted into triiodothyronine T3 it becomes the active form of the thyroid hormone and initiates metabolism, which is the process of how the body breaks down foods into smaller molecules that the body can absorb. The thyroid hormone mechanism inside the cell is to bind to the nucleus and cell receptors and starts copying DNA for producing proteins. The thyroid gland is controlled by the Pituitary gland which produces the thyroid stimulating hormone (TSH). The pituitary gland located in the brain receives information from the body through signs like metabolism, blood pressure and other signals. It responds by increasing TSH synthesis which travels to the thyroid gland increasing thyroxine production or decreasing TSH synthesis which slows the production of thyroxine. In the diagnosis of thyroid conditions, TSH levels are checked in the body. Low levels of TSH found in the body is called hypothyroidism, High levels of TSH found in the body is called hyperthyroidism. Low levels of TSH is usually treated with "synthetic TSH" in a tablet form. While high levels of TSH are treated with radioactive iodine to lower the levels.

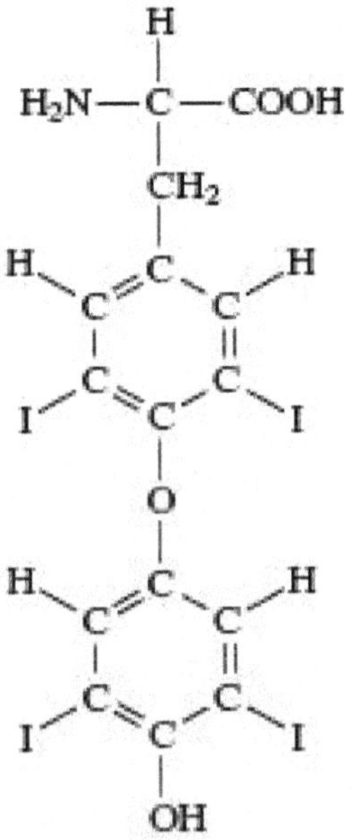

$$H_2N-\underset{\underset{\displaystyle CH_2}{|}}{\overset{\overset{\displaystyle H}{|}}{C}}-COOH$$

thyroxine (Thy)
occurs only in the hormone protein
thyroglobulin: I=iodine

Let's examine the hormone produced by the thyroid gland. For thyroxine (T4) to be made the body must have 4 Iodine atoms to bind with tyrosine which is an amino acid. The thing about Iodine and why it is so crucial is because the body cannot make this mineral. Iodine has to be ingested from our food to get in the body. If the Iodine isn't obtained every day from the food we eat the thyroid gland won't be able to make this vital hormone or its substituent triiodothyronine (T3).

**Here are some symptoms of Hypothyroidism (low Iodine)**

1) Hair loss

2) Coarse Dry hair/skin

3) Fatigue

4) Weight gain or difficulty losing weight from reduced calorie intake

5) Muscle cramps and aches

6) Decreased Libido

7) Irregular menstrual cycles

8) Constipation

9) Depression

10) Cold sensitivity

Synthetic T4 replacements are made up of a tetraiodothyronine sodium salt, which is synthetic in design but identical to the hormone created by the Thyroid gland. Some of the "inactive" ingredients are talc, magnesium stearate, confectioner's sugar (which contains corn starch) just to name a few. The interesting things are the different color additives used, like Red No. 40 Aluminum Lake and Yellow No.6 Aluminum Lake. Red 40 is a color additive found in a lot of products. It's derived from petroleum distillates or coal tars. The Center for Sciences in the Public Interest states "Red 40 and other color dyes can cause allergic reactions in some people". Studies have shown they cause hyperactivity in children and immune system tumors in rats. One ingredient in Red 40 is p-Cresidine, which is "reasonably anticipated" to be a human carcinogen as stated by the Department of Human Health Services. When taking synthetic thyroid, dosage and levels must be carefully monitored. If not some consequences are effects on development and growth, bone metabolism, gastrointestinal functions, reproductive function, emotional state and on glucose and lipid metabolism.

In women, synthetic thyroid replacement has been shown to increase bone resorption, therefore decreasing bone mineral density, in women who are post-menopausal who take higher replacement doses and in women who are receiving suppressive doses of synthetic thyroid. The increased bone resorption is likely associated with increased urinary excretion of calcium and phosphorous, as well as suppressed parathyroid hormone levels.

While taking synthetic hormone, there are other drugs that taken alongside that can cause a Drug to Drug interaction. These drugs may decrease T4 absorption and result in hypothyroidism.

- Antacids (Aluminum and Magnesium)

- Ferrous Sulfate

- Calcium Carbonate

- Hydroxides (Simethicone)

Iodine is a mineral that cannot be created inside the body. It must be ingested with food or other supplements. The thyroid needs at least 70 mcg of Iodine to synthesize thyroxine (T4) and triiodothyronine (T3). Iodine is crucial for children as it facilitates both physical and mental growth. A sufficient amount of iodine promotes the development of basic skills such as language, movement, and hearing. Iodine is important for overall IQ. The average adult needs around 150 micrograms a day. Infants up to 12 months need around 120 micrograms a day. Children up to 8 years old need around 80 micrograms, from 13 years up the suggested amount is 130 micrograms. Women who are pregnant and those breastfeeding need 220 and 290 micrograms a day respectively. In adults, the agreed amount for maximum intake is 1,000 micrograms a day

## Electric/Alkaline herb for thyroid

- Bladderwrack (Fucus vesiculosus) - has the most iodine that is found in nature. Bladderwrack is made up of iodine, calcium, magnesium, potassium, sodium, silicon, iron, B-complex vitamins minerals, trace metals, phenolics, algin, lipids and phlorotannins. Other constituents are Vitamin A,C,E,K,S and G. Bladderwrack has been used traditionally to treat thyroid conditions. One capsule of Bladderwrack supplements can contain up to 600 micrograms per gram of natural Iodine.

## TCM herb for thyroid

- Panax Ginseng one of the most known herbs of all time is often used. In TCM, with the thyroid gland being part of the endocrine system as well as connected to the pituitary gland a Yang Herb is best suited. Panax

Ginseng is said to replace and replenish lost Ch'i in the energy meridians and organs. Panax Ginseng originates from China, Japan, or Korea. The name Panax is derived from the Greek word "panacea" which translates to 'cure all' or 'remedy for all disease'. Panax ginseng has a sweet and slightly bitter flavor. One constituent of Panax Ginseng is Panaquilon, which is an endocrine tonic and has regulatory effects on the endocrine system, most likely in the hypothalamus and pituitary gland which manufacture TSH.

## Ayurveda/Rasayana herb for thyroid

- Ashwagandha (Withania somnifera)-, also known as Indian Ginseng shows very promising effects on the thyroid. From an Auryvedic to much sweet ras and an imbalance in Pitta is correlated to an imbalance of the endocrine system. In studies on mice, they were given ashwagandha and their thyroid hormones were observed. The treatment raised T3 levels by 18% and T4 levels by 111% after just 20 days. In human studies patients treated with Ashwagandha saw an improvement of TSH, as well as raised levels of T4 from baseline up to 24%.

- Guggul (Commiphora Mukul). According to scientists, Guggul helps fight against low performing thyroid function by enhancing the conversion of T4 to T3, which is a more potent form of the thyroid hormone. About 80% T4 and 20% T3 are manufactured in the thyroid gland. Most of the T3 is made in the peripheral tissues by the conversion of T4 to T3. T3 has about 4 times the hormone strength as T4.

## Foods for thyroid

- Kelp, Dulse, Nori, Wakame and Sea moss are some examples of sea vegetables. Cranberries are a good source as well. Roughly 4 ounces of cranberries contain 400 micrograms of Iodine, best to get organic if possible. One medium sized organic potato with the skin left on has about 60 micrograms of iodine.

# Chapter 5: Hypertension

Before the early 1900's high blood pressure wasn't a specific "disease". There wasn't a sphygmometer (a device that measures blood pressure) invented yet. All people knew was the symptoms associated with Hypertension and how to treat it. Some of the symptoms where: Obesity, Diabetes, Erectile Dysfunction, Kidney Disease and heart disease to name a few. So how exactly is blood pressure measured?

## A sphygmometer

| BP category | Systolic | | Diastolic |
|---|---|---|---|
| | mm Hg (upper#) | | mm Hg (lower #) |
| | | | |
| Normal | Less than 120 | and | Less than 120 |
| Prehypertension | 120-139 | or | 80-89 |
| High BP, Stage 1 hypertension | 140-150 | or | 90-100 |
| High BP, Stage 2 hypertension | 160 or greater | or | 100 or greater |
| Hypertensive Crisis | 180 or greater | or | 110 or greater |

The blood pressure in the body is constantly changing. You can test ten different times and get different readings. In general, it's best to test 2 to3 times in the morning for a week and take the average of those roughly. Another indicator of hypertension is the pulse rate of the heart. A normal pulse rate is 60-100 Beats Per Minute. The range of 70-80 is considered normal. While anything above 80 Beats Per Minute is usually a sign of HBP.

When the heart beats pressure in the arteries increases which equals the Systolic pressure (upper #) between beats, pressure in the arteries decreases which equals diastolic pressure (lower #)

**The heart has 4 chambers:**

- The Right atrium, which receives blood from the veins and pumps it into the right ventricle.

- The right ventricle receives the blood from the right atrium and pumps it into the lungs where it's oxygenated.

- The Left atrium, which receives oxygenated blood from the lungs and pumps it into the left ventricle.

- The Left ventricle (the strongest chamber) pumps oxygenated blood to the rest of the body. The left ventricle's intense contractions create our blood pressure.

There are coronary arteries that are on the surface of the heart which provide oxygenated blood to the heart muscle. A web-like connection of nerve tissues runs throughout the heart, conducting the signals that govern contraction and relaxation. Surrounding the heart is a sac called the pericardium, which in TCM is associated with the Circulation-sex meridian.

Primary hypertension is responsible for 85% to 90% of diagnosed hypertension, often called the lifestyle disease. These causes are usually things that can be adjusted without drugs and often without herbs but with a diet and lifestyle rearrangement. Secondary hypertension is generally associated with the younger population. Most times kidney, endocrine system and other birth defects are the catalyst for secondary hypertension.

## Causes of High Blood Pressure

- Blood pressure increases with age blood vessels aren't as pliable as we age; could lead to atherosclerosis.

- A potassium and Vitamin D deficiency

- Heavy Salt (Sodium) intake

- Overweight people tend to have higher occurrence of HBP

- Varying in Hormones can affect BP levels

- If the Kidney's aren't functioning properly, can lead to HBP

- Stress and Anxiety can cause spikes in BP

- Genetics can be a factor

- Race (African Americans) are at a higher risk to develop Hypertension

- Diabetics experience more instances of HBP

- Smokers are more likely to have HBP over non-smokers

**A general Diagnosis of any 4 of the below is often used to Identify Hypertension:**

1) Shortness of Breath

2) Dizziness

3) Palpations or increases heart beats

4) Trembling

5) Sweating

6) Nausea or stomach upset

7) Numbness, tingling

8) Hot or cold flashes

9) Chest pains

10) Fear of dying or fear of going crazy

## HBP- The Silent Killer

- Hypertension is suggested as either the primary or contributing cause of death for at least 1000 people a day in the United States.

- HBP is the leading cause of stroke

- HBP is the major precipitating cause of Heart attacks

- 69% of people who have had their first heart attack, 77% of people who have their first stroke and 74% who have heart failure also have HBP.

- In the United States, 1 out of 3 (31%) of the adult population has high blood pressure. That's at least 80 million people, which only half of these have their HBP under control.

- Another 30% of the population has prehypertension

**The conventional treatment for HBP includes:**

1) Diuretics- increase the kidneys mechanism of action, by promoting excess water to be excreted. The prolonged use of diuretics to manage HBP severely depletes the body of essential minerals. Some of the minerals that can be excreted in the fluids from the body are magnesium, potassium, sodium, chloride, zinc, and iodine. Diuretics block the kidney's ability to reabsorb these minerals, especially sodium.

2) Alpha-adrenergic blockers and Beta blockers –Alpha and Beta blockers were designed to weaken the heart and relax the blood vessels. Beta blockers work by eliminating the ability of the heart to respond to

epinephrine and adrenaline, which stimulates the pulse rate of the heart and blood pressure increasing both. By design, these drugs were meant to "weaken" the heart so blood pressure is reduced and heart pain reduced.

3) Calcium channel blockers, Ace inhibitors And Angiotensin II receptor blockers – decrease blood pressure by blocking the pathway of Calcium into the arterial wall cells. This action causes the vessels to become more relaxed as less constricted. Calcium is needed in the body for a variety of cardiovascular functions, contraction mechanism of the heart and smooth muscle, and for storage and use of energy in cells. Calcium blockers shouldn't be taken for an extended period of time. Anything that overrides your body natural function and blocks the use of such an important mineral isn't beneficial in the long run.

Most times several of these types of drugs are prescribed simultaneously in the treatment of HBP.

## Common Adverse Reaction to Antihypertensive Diuretics

- Menstrual Inconsistency

- Sexual dysfunction

- Gastrointestinal problems

- Nausea

- Glucose intolerance

- Hypokalemia

- Hypercholesterolemia

- Gynecomastia

## Common Adverse Reaction of Alpha and Beta Blockers

- Sexual dysfunction

- Insomnia

- Fatigue

- Decreased HDL cholesterol

- Bronchospasm

- Increases chances of heart failure

- Masking of hyperglycemia

Common Adverse Reactions of Calcium channel blockers, ACE inhibitors and Angiotensin II Receptor Blockers

- Rash

- Sexual dysfunction

- Angioedema

- Headache

- Hyperkalemia

The Number needed to treat for people with mild hypertension and no pre-existing cardiovascular disease who took blood pressure medicines for five years to prevent death, cardiovascular death, and strokes: 1 in 111 for the risk of overall death

1 in 82 for cardiovascular death

1 in 172 for a stroke

For the number needed to harm of people on anti-hypertensive medications for five years was:

1 in 10 was harmed (experienced side effects, discontinued medication).

Hypertension is not a single disease, but a symptom of other factors that are hidden. That's why Hypertension is known as the "silent killer". Conventional treatment of hypertension is to lower and maintain control of the body's blood pressure by "lessening" the effectiveness of the heart, the uptake and use of minerals, and by blocking the body's natural mechanisms. In TCM some causes of Hypertension are:

1) Constitution –

2) Excess Yang – hyper-achiever, go-getter. Expels a lot of Yang (heat)

3) Insufficient Yin- people with excess Yang have less Yin (cool) energy in them. Yang is equivalent to a motor in a car, and Yin is like the oil that runs in the motor

4) Diet- you are what you eat

5) Insufficient exercise

6) Not enough rest- Melatonin the "sleep hormone" may

7) Stress

## TCM herbs for hypertension

- **Hibiscus (Hibiscus sabdariffa),** which is used in TCM and Auryvedic practice, is a highly effective anti-hypertensive herb. It has been compared to ACE inhibitors like Lisinopril and Captopril. Hibiscus has diuretic properties, the less volume in the blood the lower the pressure also by acting as a natural ACE inhibitor it relaxes the small arteries and capillary systems of the heart (Nwachukwu DC, 2015). Approximately 1/3 of the blood is located in the arteries, easing tension there will lower blood pressure. According to scientific research 2 to 3 cups a day of hibiscus tea is needed for a therapeutic dose. One study found hibiscus tea to be as effective if not greater in treating mild to moderate hypertension than hydrochlorothiazide (HCTZ). Unlike HCTZ which can alter the electrolyte balance in the body, hibiscus did not.

- **Eucommia bark/Tu Chung (Eucommia ulmoides)** - A kidney Yang tonic, used to treat kidneys and liver meridians in the body. In clinical trials, eucommia bark was shown to have blood pressure lowering constituents which acts like a natural beta-adrenergic blocker to help dilate blood vessels (Greenway F, 2011). Eucommia has been shown to have a rich source of amino acids, vitamins, minerals, and flavonoids. Flavonoids are compounds that are found in nature and considered as secondary metabolites and function as chemical messengers, normal body function regulations and cell cycle inhibitors. A total of 7 different flavonoids have been isolated from eucommia. The great thing about this herb are no known drug interactions are side effects.

- **Hawthorne berries (Crataegus) -** are also used in treatment for hypertension. Hawthorne promotes blood flow into smaller vessels. Hawthorne acts as a natural ACE inhibitor, Calcium blocker and Nitric Oxide release (vasodilator) to reduce blood pressure and halt the manufacturing of angiotensin II, a blood vessel dilator in charge of increasing blood pressure. Hawthorne is food for senile hearts, hypertensive hearts, weakness of the myocardium, cardiac arrhythmias, and angina. * Not for use of pregnant women, or people taking Warfarin (may increase anti-coagulation).

In Ayurveda (Rasayana) hypertension is described as Rakta Gata Vata. Rakta Gata Vata is essentially a disorder of the blood caused by excess vata and pitta. The kapha will also be affected leading to loss and support of cardiovascular functions. In Ayurveda vata is located in the colon, toxin's in the colon can be absorbed into the blood and cause constrictions in the blood vessels, especially the arteries. Vata in the colon is dry and cold which ultimately leads to constipation. Hypertension in vata could be increased due to mental anxiety, stress and worries in general. The small intestines in Ayurveda are the location of pitta in the body. Toxins from undigested food in the intestines which move through the circulation of the body. The toxins cause the blood to be viscous, this increased viscosity causes the blood to add pressure on the blood vessels. In pitta, hypertension could be increased by strong emotions like fear, anger, and jealousy. Kapha is located in the stomach in Ayurveda, Kapha like gastric secretions are involved in the digestion of carbohydrates, starch, and glucose. The end product of this phase of digestion is triglycerides. When Kapha in the stomach is disturbed there is an increase in triglycerides and cholesterol (which is another form of kapha). The blood becomes thicker and causes fatty molecules to deposit in the blood vessels, which leads to narrowing of the arteries and a possible heart attack. Hypertension in kapha could be due to factors of malfunctioning of internal vital organs (liver, heart, kidneys, etc).

## Ayurveda/Rasayana herbs for hypertension

- **Ashwagandha (Withania somnifera)** also known as Indian Ginseng has been used in Ayurveda since ancient times. Ashwagandha is used by the body to reduce stress due to its mild sedative action on the body. This anti-stress quality is why it is used for hypertension. Has been shown to restore stress-induced depletion of the adrenals. Ashwagandha is used as a natural calcium channel blocker as well as a beta blocker and is able to reduce systolic blood pressure. Calcium dilates the heart, too much calcium in the body keeps the heart contracted and not relaxed.

- **Arjuna (Terminalia arjuna)** is an Ayurveda herb used to treat hypertension as well. Arjuna bark is rich with natural antioxidants (flavonoids), saponins, coenzyme Q-10, and minerals like magnesium, zinc, copper, and calcium. Co-enzyme Q-10 is a molecule essential for ATP, which provides energy to all cells. The body can make co-enzyme 10 but production starts to deteriorate around 50 years old. The heart muscle cells require a lot of metabolic energy to function properly, especially since they are always working. The clinical benefits of coenzyme Q10 are many it can improve energy production, act as an antioxidant, and stabilize membrane fluidity, decreasing blood viscosity, thereby improving hypertension. Also, if you suffer from cardiovascular ailments or just want to keep your heart function at a healthy level, you may wish to consider supplementing your diet with coenzyme Q10. Coenzyme Q- 10 is also great for heart health has been shown to help prevent heart attacks. Arjuna acts like a natural beta blocker in the body and has been clinically tested to raise the systolic pressure in the body. Has mild diuretic properties, lower blood lipid levels, help reduce blood clot formation.

- **Tulsi/ Holy Basil (Ocimum sanctum)** is one of the foundation herbs in Ayurvedic practice, often called "The Queen of herbs" or an "Elixir of Life". Used to neutralize kapha and to balance pitta and vata in the body. Holy Basil is considered an adaptogen, a herb that increases the body response to stress. Flavonoids, tannins, essential oils, calcium, iron, chlorophyll, zinc, manganese, sodium, vitamins A and C are found in Holy Basil. As a rich source of Magnesium, which relaxes the heart, holy basil has been shown to have blood pressure lowering effects. In a study on animals, holy basil lowered systolic blood pressure by 20 mmHg and lowered diastolic blood pressure by 15 mmHg over a 4 week period.

- **Winter Melon (Ash Gourd)** is used in the Ayurvedic system of healing as a medicinal food. Classified as a vegetable and not a fruit, it's the only species of Benincasa hispida genus. Some constituents are a high concentration of Vitamin C and B2, zinc, iron potassium, phosphorous, calcium, niacin, thiamine and some amino acids. The rind has been shown to possess diuretic properties, which helps the body to get expel toxins and lower blood pressure. With its high level of Potassium, winter melon is very effective in cardiovascular health maintenance. Potassium acts as a vasodilator, meaning it can lower blood pressure by releasing tension that has built up in the blood vessels and arteries, allowing blood to flow more freely.

## Electric/Alkaline Herbs

**Cayenne Pepper (Capsicum Annum)** is on Dr. Sebi nutritional guide list as an alkaline seasoning alternative. Cayenne Pepper has a blood moving effect on the body which causes the warm sensation when digested. The cayenne pepper has Vitamin A, Vitamin B6, Vitamin E, Vitamin C, Vitamin B2, potassium and manganese. One of Cayenne Pepper active ingredients is capsaicin, which has been found to drop systemic blood pressure. Cayenne Pepper has been shown to have natural ACE inhibitor effects on blood pressure.

**Valerian Root (Valeriana officinalis)** is used as a sedative and a sleep aid. It helps relaxes the body and combats stress. By lowering stress in the body and its sedative nature, it has been shown to lower blood pressure as well. Valerian root is made up of calcium, iron, magnesium, manganese, potassium, zinc, selenium, B Vitamins, Vitamin C and essential fatty acids. Also made up of phytonutrients like Beta- Carotene, which is a powerhouse antioxidant excellent for cardiovascular health and Limonene, which falls under the classification as terpenes. Limonene is found in the oil of citrus peels. Research has shown that limonene can enable apoptosis (death signal) that terminates cancer cells and keep them from reproducing. Limonene also raises the level of enzymes in the liver that can detoxify carcinogens in the body.

**Soursop (Guanabana)** is a native fruit of South America. Soursop has amino acids, Vitamin B, Vitamin C, iron, folate, Vitamin E, Vitamin k, selenium, potassium and zinc. The stems of the bark also contain Co Q-10, which has been shown to lower both systolic and diastolic blood pressure in the human body. In animal studies, Soursop was effective as a vasodilator (relaxes the tension on the blood vessels and arteries) and has hypotensive (low blood pressure) properties. The high amounts of potassium found in Soursop are very beneficial, potassium helps reduce the effects of sodium in the body.

## Foods that help lower blood pressure

- **Olive leaf extract** is a good natural alternative for hypertension. Olive leaf extract contains flavonoids and triterpenes. One of the main phytonutrients is Oleuropein which is a Polyphenol. Oleuropein is a powerful antioxidant, it has been shown to act like a natural vasodilator allowing for better blood flow, and also by being such a powerful antioxidant, it gets rid of free radicals in the body. Free radicals can cause inflammation of the blood vessels and arteries which alternatively LDL cholesterol can attach to the inflamed areas. This can cause the blood vessels and arteries to narrow thus increasing blood pressure. Olive leaf was tested to be as effective as pharmaceutical drug Captopril a synthetic ACE inhibitor.

- **Watercress (Nasturtium Officinale)** is a green, leafy vegetable that grows naturally by spring water.

Research has shown that watercress is the most nutrient dense vegetables on this planet. Watercress contains Vitamins A,C,B1,B6,E,K as well as folic acid, calcium, iodine, iron, manganese, phosphorous, zinc, magnesium, plus phytonutrients: beta-carotene, lutein, quercetin and glucosinolate. The phytonutrient lutein, normally good for eye health has shown to also lower blood pressure, by reducing arterial wall thickening which leads to poor blood flow. One cup of raw watercress has over 100% requirement a day of Vitamin K alone. With its high mineral content especially calcium and magnesium which are synergistic in their role in regulating blood pressure, watercress is a vegetable that should be added to anyone's diet.

# Chapter 6: Diabetes

To understand Diabetes and what it is we have to start at the Pancreas. As part of the endocrine system, the pancreas is an organ located in the abdominal region of the body. The pancreas sits behind the stomach and attaches to the small intestines. The pancreas has 2 vital roles in the body, first, it aids in digestion. When food reaches the top of the small intestines, the pancreas produces a substance filled with enzymes which start to break down the food. Secondly, the pancreas helps regulate blood sugar levels in the body by producing hormones. The blood glucose (sugar) levels must be maintained at certain ratios in the body. There must be a constant supply of sugar to feed the cells but not too much so that the kidneys and other organs are negatively affected. The pancreas manufactures 2 hormones to help maintain the blood sugar: Glucagon, which raises glucose levels by stimulating the liver to metabolize glucose into glucose molecules which are released in the blood. The other hormone is Insulin: this hormone lowers blood glucose after a meal by stimulating the absorption of glucose by the liver along with muscles and fat tissues.

Diabetes is classified as either diabetes mellitus or diabetes insipidus. When in reference to diabetes, most people are refereeing to diabetes mellitus. Diabetes insipidus is a rare, uncommon disorder. Diabetes mellitus is broken into 2 categories: type 1 (insulin dependent) and type 2 (non-insulin dependent).

## Let's look at how insulin plays a role in the body

Food is broken down into 3 different categories proteins, fats and carbohydrates. Out of the three carbohydrates raises blood sugar levels in the body the fastest. Carbohydrates are made of sugar starch. When carbohydrates are eaten especially those low in fiber, insulin is released so it can carry glucose into the cells. The cells have insulin receptor sites attached to them which allow the cell to absorb the glucose and make energy. This bodily process can only happen at a certain rate so the excess glucose has to be stored somewhere else in the body. In the form of glycogen, the body can hold up to 200 grams of glucose in the muscles and 70 grams of glucose in the liver. When those two places have filled up the insulin receptors decrease on those cells so glucose won't go in. The excess glucose has to go somewhere and one of the worst places is in the bloodstream. When glucose gets into the bloodstream it starts to bind to proteins in a process called glycation. Glycation is a process where sugar in the bloodstream attaches to proteins, lipids or nucleic acid and creates Advanced Glycation Endproducts (AGE). An example in Nature would be the ripening of a banana. Over a time dark spots start to appear on a banana that is sweet, the same thing happens in the body in the presence of AGE. AGE's or known as glycotoxins, which in abundance in the body can lead to diabetes, hypertension and other chronic diseases. The problem with the excess AGE's in the body especially in diabetics lies in the ability for these glycotoxins to get into the bloodstream and capillaries. A lot of diabetics can lose sight or have a leg, feet or toes amputated because these are the sites with very small arteries where it's easy for the glycotoxins to get stuck and cause a lot of damage.

Once the body has stored all the glucose in the muscles and liver and doesn't want the excess glycation process to happen it decreases the insulin receptors on most cells not allowing glucose to get in. The extra glucose gets broken down and converted to triglycerides and gets stored in the only place that the insulin cell receptors are actually increasing and that's the fat cells of the body!! Wherever there is insulin there will be fat, they go hand in hand. To use the energy stored in our fat tissues, fatty acids are taken out of the tissue to be broken down for energy thus making you lose fat. But when the insulin levels are too high you cannot break down your fat tissues. The enzyme that allows fatty acids to be broken down from stored fat is Hormone Sensitive Lipase, which is insulin sensitive and will not allow the fat to be broken down when in the presence of insulin. When there is too much insulin in the body you can't burn stored fat, thus you always feel hungry and feel lethargic. The only fuel the body can burn is more glucose causing you to eat more and more to replace the energy, which causes you to get fat.

Sucrose (table sugar) is made up of one part fructose and one part glucose. Sucrose is in over 80% of the products in the grocery store. Diabetes is known as sugar in the blood like we learned before carbohydrates are sugars and starch. The body treats fructose identical to the way it treats alcohol, as a toxin. Whenever we inject something with fructose in it at least 90% gets metabolized by the liver, by bypassing the normal metabolic route and going directly to the liver, fructose is converted into pyruvate then to citrate which is then converted to VLDL (low-density lipoprotein). VLDL leads to fat accumulation in the abdomen area (beer belly, soda belly). Some of the citrates is converted to Free Fatty Acids as well and can get into the muscles of the body and cause muscle insulin resistance. Not all citrate is able to escape the liver, which can cause fat deposits in the liver known as fatty liver disease. Fructose also produces Uric Acid when metabolized, which causes high blood pressure and leads to hypertension.

| Type 1 Diabetes | Type 2 diabetes |
| --- | --- |
| Destroys the beta cells in the pancreas, thus the pancreas cannot produce insulin. | The ineffective use of insulin on the body and is known as insulin resistance |
| Not associated with excess body weight | Associated with excess body weight |
| Autoimmune disease | Low sensitivity to insulin. Insulin isn't reducing glucose levels as it should |
| Everyone with type 1 diabetes has to inject insulin, therefore insulin dependent | Often need insulin injection to avoid hyperglycemia( high blood sugar) |
| Higher ketone levels at initial diagnosis | Treated with medications and injections. Possible to control |

When using the word diabetes, we often refer to type 2, diabetes related to type 1 being a rare condition.

**Different classifications of the most prescribed type 2 diabetes are**

- **Thiazolidinediones (Actos)** – target the PPAR gamma receptors which play a role in how the body stores fat and metabolizes glucose. They can cause the body to keep extra fluid, which can cause swelling (edema) and weight gain. The extra fluid can worsen or lead to heart failure. Some other side effects: bladder cancer, broken bones, diabetic eye disease with swelling in the back of the eye (macular edema), liver problems, sore throat, muscle pain, upper respiratory infections.

- **Sulfonylureas (Glimperide)** – sulfonylureas bind to the beta cells in the pancreas to increase the amount of insulin produced. Some side effects are Weight gain (wherever there is insulin, there is fat), hypoglycemia (low blood pressure)

- **Sodium-glucose transporter (SGLT) 2 inhibitors (invokana)** – affects the kidney's ability to reabsorb glucose back into the blood, thus lowering blood glucose levels. The body expels the excess glucose through the urine. Can cause hypoglycemia (low blood pressure), urinary tract infections (excess glucose going thru the urine) and possibly liver damage as well.

- **DPP-4 inhibitors (Januvia)** – blocks the body's natural enzyme DDP-4. DDP-4 is an enzyme found in almost every cell, it plays a role in immune response, mediates cell to cell interactions and apoptosis (bad cell death). DDP-4 also blocks intestinal hormones called incretins, incretins stimulate insulin and reduce glycogen in the liver. Can cause pancreatitis (inflamed pancreas), skin reactions, flu-like symptoms and intestinal problems.

- **Biguanides (metformin)** – work by blocking the liver ability to make glucose from amino acids and proteins, also by activating an enzyme (AMPK) which allows cells to respond more efficiently to insulin and metabolize glucose in the blood. Biguanides like metformin have been shown to cause lactic acidosis. Lactic acidosis is the buildup of lactate (L-lactate) in the kidneys which drastically lowers the body's pH. Biguanides cause an increase in production and decrease in the removal of lactate leading to elevated cellular lactate levels. Also can cause loss of b 12, flatulence, diarrhea, sleepiness and muscle and joint pain.

The reported number needed to treat for type 2 diabetes for over 5 years of treatment with prescription medications were: none were helped (prevented stroke), none were helped (prevented death), none were helped( prevented heart attack), none were helped prevented kidney failure) and 1 in 250 were helped (prevented limb amputation)

The reported number needed to harm was 1 in 6 over 5 years (severe hypoglycemia hospitalization required).

## TCM Diabetes

In Traditional Chinese Medicine Diabetes is referred to as Xiao-ke "wasting and thirsting". Diabetes is divided into three parts of the organ-meridian system: upper, middle and lower. The upper type of diabetes is characterized by excessive thirst, the middle is associated with excessive hunger and the lower by excessive urination. Ironically those are the clinical symptoms for the diagnosis of diabetes from the western approach. The Triple Warmer in TCM is a Yang fire organ meridian function. The Triple Warmer is responsible for the manufacturing of "essential energy" which has 2 different types: the nourishment aspect is "Ying Ch'i" (blood) which flows through the meridians and the protective aspect "Wei Ch'i" (lymph fluid) which flows into the muscles, joints, skin and bones and protects the body against attacks from external forces. The Triple Warmer's general location in the body is in the throat, abdomen, and pelvic region. The Upper burning harmonizes the lung and heart meridians and moves the essential energy Ying and Wei. The middle burning harmonizes the stomach and spleen, so it's responsible for nutrient removal from food and the digestion of food. The lower burning harmonizes the liver, kidney, intestine, and bladder area and is responsible for the intake of nutrients, elimination of waste, storage of energy and reproductive functions. With the triple warmer system being a Yang aspect, Yin deficiency is often associated with Diabetes (Xiao-ke) in TCM. Yin deficiency signs are fatigue, weakness, lethargy and a pale complexion. The other two factors in a Xiao-ke diagnosis are improper diet (large amounts of sweets, carbohydrates, greasy, fried foods, alcohol and hot drinks) and emotional stress (worry, anxiety, depression).

## TCM herbs for Diabetes

- **Chinese Cucumber/ Trichosanthes Root (Tian Hua Fen)** has been used for thousands of years for its cooling effects. Diabetes is said to be heat in the body, so this balances out the heat. Chinese Cucumber is sweet, its essence cold, it enters the lung and stomach meridians. Its function is to clear heat and halt excessive thirst, increase stomach and intestinal fluids. The main function is treating yin deficiency and middle burning diabetes. In countries like China and Taiwan, trichosanthes is the most widely used herb to treat diabetes. Trichosanthes have proven to have shown hypoglycemic in animal test as well as the ability to improve glucose tolerance.

- **Poria/ Fu Ling (Poria cocos)** is a medicinal mushroom long used in TCM. One of the most widely used herbs for Yin. For being a Yin herb, which is great for fluid retention, Poria regulates metabolism and enhances the bladder and kidneys. Also helps the movement of Ch'i of the Triple Warmer, which is essential to the vital meridians. In animal studies with type 2 diabetes, poria showed hypoglycemic effect. One of the ingredients in Poria, dehydrotrametenolic acid was shown to affect the PPA R gamma receptor (which is involved in insulin sensitivity) like a natural version of Thiazolidinediones.

- **Chinese Licorice Root/ Kan Tsao (Glycyrrhizae uralensis)** is the most widely used herb in China. Beneficial for all 12 meridians especially to the Spleen, Stomach, and Lungs. Chinese licorice has been attributed with balancing the middle burning center part of the triple warmer meridians. Known as the great detoxifier, Chinese licorice cleans the body and blood of excess toxins. Because of its detoxifying attributes, Chinese licorice has been used to regulate blood sugar levels in the body. One of the compounds in Chinese licorice is isoliquiritigenin, which was shown to help prevent high fat, lifestyle-related obesity, fatty liver disease and type 2 diabetes by stopping activation of NLRP3, a protein associated with Diabetes.

## Ayurveda/ Rasayana Diabetes

The term that correlates with diabetes in Ayurveda text is Prameha, 'pra' meaning abundance and 'meha' meaning urine. Prameha is characterized by excessive urination (in frequency and quantity) and turbidity (the cloudiness of a fluid by large numbers of sediments). All 3 doshas vata, pitta, and kapha are affected by Prameha. In the first stage, Kapha (which governs bile and fat and is disturbed by excess sweets like carbohydrates) is in excess thereby precipitating Kaphaja Prameha (pre-diabetes). Further progression leads to a loss of Kapha. Pitta then predominates, which governs the blood, leads to Pittaja Prameha (acute diabetes). Further progression leads to losing of Pitta. This ends with Vata, which carries vital substances out of the body through the urine, leading to Vataja Prameha (chronic diabetes).

## Signs of Prameha

| Kaphaja | Pittaja | Vataja |
| --- | --- | --- |
| Stuffy nose | Excessive thirst | Excessive hunger |
| laziness | fever | Heaviness in the chest |
| anorexia | anemia | insomnia |
| Excessive salivation | Pain in the penis or bladder areas | tremors |
| vomiting | Burning sensations | pain |
| cough | diarrhea | constipation |
| indigestion | Too much acid accumulation | Dyspnea (shortness of breath) |

**In Ayurveda there are 3 different types of Prameha (Diabetes):**

1) Prabhuta Mootrata- prameha associated with frequency of urination.

2) Avila Mootrata- prameha associated with turbidity (cloudiness) of urine.

3) Madhumeha- associated with glucose (sugar) in the urine.

There are about 20 different pathways that Prameha are classified for in the body through the flow of urine. Each of these pathways has a name and effects the 3 doshas. Kapha has 10 different pramehas, Pitta has 6 different pramehas, and Vata has 4 different pramehas.

**Kapha (pre diabetes) Prameha:**

| Name of Prameha | Equivalent name | Signs in the urine |
|---|---|---|
| Udakameha | Hydruria | Urine is colorless like water, excessive flow, feels cold |
| Ikshuvalikameha | Glycosuria | Urine contains sugar, cloudy in color, |

| | | |
|---|---|---|
| | | sweet, resembles sugar water |
| Sandrameha | Chyluria | If the lymphatic flow is disrupted chyle can leak into the kidneys and urine, causing urine to appear white like milk. Urine very viscous. |
| Sandra Prasadmeha | Belluria | Urine is slightly diluted with glucose, semi-viscous |
| Shukrameha | No equivalent name | Urine appears chalky white in color, body hairs are excited while passing urine |
| Shukrameha | Spermaturia | Urine contains sperm, urine appears thick |
| Sheetameha | Phosturia | Urine is white and cold and sweet to taste |
| Siktameha | Graveluria | Sand like particles in urine, sign of renal stones |
| Shanairmeha | Oliguria | Urine flow becomes slow and output is difficult |
| Lalameha | Pyuria | Urine contains white blood cells or pus, sign of UTI, urine gum like |

## Pitta (acute diabetes) Prameha:

| Name of Prameha | Equivalent name | Signs in the urine |
|---|---|---|
| Kalameha | Melanuria | Urine contains melanin, urine appears from orange to black in color |
| Nilameha | Indigouria | Urine appears blue in color |
| Raktameha | Hematuria | Blood in the urine, urine appears red in color |
| Manjishthameha | Hemoglobinuria | Urine appears pink in color, urine is foul smelling |
| Haridrameha | Urobilinuria | Urine is yellow in color, pungent smell may feel burning sensations |
| Ksharmeha | Alkaluria | Urine which is slightly acidic is now more alkaline |

## Vata (Chronic Diabetes) Prameha:

| Name of Prameha | Equivalent name | Signs in the urine |
|---|---|---|
| Vasameha | Lipuria | Urine is yellowish in color, urine contains lipids (fats/vasa) |

| Majjameha | Myelouria | Urine contains bone marrow (majja), urine looks like nerve tissues. |
|---|---|---|
| Hastimeha | Diabetes insipidus | Urine volume is extremely large, urine contains lymph (lasika) |
| Madhumeha | Diabetes Mellitus (type 2) | Urine is cloudy, sweet, and pale in color, essence of the body (Oja) is loss |

A perfect example of the correlation of Ayurveda and the body would be the Pitta Prameha Haridrameha (Urobilinuria). In the body urobolin (a chemical that gives urine its yellowish color) is manufactured in the intestinal tract. Urobolin is a byproduct from Bilirubin, which is produced when the liver breaks down old red blood cells. Bilrubin is located in bile and is brownish/yellowish in color. Urobilinuria is a result of the inability of the liver cells to filter from circulation the urobilin brought to the liver by the blood. Urobolin passes into the circulation of the kidneys and is expelled in the urine. If too much urobilin accumulates in the intestines damage to the liver can occur. Now we can see how this is a Pitta imbalance, Pitta governs the blood and its functions in Ayurveda philosophy. If the blood and liver aren't working properly a clear sign is yellowish urine being expelled.

## Ayurveda/Rasayana herbs for Diabetes

- **Fenugreek (Trigonella foenum-graecum)** is not a seed but a legume that has been used in Ayurveda medicinal practice and as a spice in kitchens in India for ages. The remains of fenugreek seeds have been even been found in the remains of buried Egyptians within the pyramids. Fenugreek slows down the absorption of glucose and other simple carbohydrates from its high fiber content. A study on the effect of fenugreek seeds on patients with type 2 diabetes had promising results. The fenugreek seeds were soaked in hot water and given over an 8 week period. The FBS level (fasting blood glucose), TG level (triglycerides), and VLDL-C level (very low-density lipoprotein cholesterol) were decreased (25%, 30%, and 365% respectively) (Kassaian N, 2009). Fenugreek seeds are high in iron, potassium, calcium, selenium, copper, zinc, manganese, magnesium, niacin, all b vitamins except B12, and Vitamins A and C. Also has polysaccharides such as saponins, tannins, hemicellulose, mucilage and pectin, these have been shown to lower LDL by stopping bile salts from absorbing in the colon. Fenugreek contains the amino acid 4 –hydroxyisoleucene which lowers the rate of glucose intake in the intestines thereby lowers blood sugar levels in patients with diabetes.

- **Indian plum/ Jamun (Syzygium jambolensis)** – Jamun is a seasonal fruit found in India and Asia. Jamun has been used treat Diabetes in Ayurveda for centuries. Jamun contains carotene, iron, folic acid, calcium, potassium, magnesium, phosphorus, antioxidants, phytonutrients, and Vitamin C. The seeds contain glucoside jamboline and ellagic acid which inhibits the conversion of starch into sugar thus controlling blood sugar levels (J. Giri, 1985). Also, has 4 times the Vitamin C as an orange. Vitamin C is a powerful antioxidant and reduces LDL from the body, which plays a role in Diabetes.

- **Bitter Gourd (Karela)/ Bitter Melon (Momordica charantia)** – is part of the Cucurbitaceae family and is indigenous to Asia, South America, India, and East Africa. Bitter Gourd reduces violated Kapha and Pitta doshas. The taste is bitter and pungent hence the name of the vegetable. One cup of bitter melon has over 140% of the recommended daily amount of Vitamin C. Bitter melon also contains zinc, potassium, magnesium, manganese, iron, copper, calcium, folate, all B vitamins except B12 as well as Vitamin A. One of the phytonutrients found in bitter melon is polypeptide-P which has been shown to lower glucose levels in animals and humans when ingested (Tayyab F, 2012). This plant "insulin" works by mimicking the action of insulin in the body which lowers blood sugar in the body. Bitter melon also contains Charantin which is a molecule only found in the plant kingdom. Charantin raises glucose absorption and glycogen production in the cells of the liver, muscles and fatty tissue. After an 8 week study on mice with type 2 diabetes who were treated with bitter melon, the results showed a significant decline in non- fasting blood glucose, plasma glucose intolerance, and insulin resistance. (Hsien-Yi Wang, 2014)

## Electric/ Alkaline herbs for Diabetes

- **Huereque/ Coyote Melon (Ibervillea sonorae)** is used in South America to treat Diabetes. Coyote melon belongs to the Cucurbitaceae or Gourd family of vegetables and is related to the cucumber. The coyote melon contains beneficial phytonutrients and tannins. One phytonutrient that is abundant in the coyote melon is Gallic Acid. Gallic acid is an acid found in plants and acts as a natural antioxidant. Gallic acid has shown in testing to have positive effects on glucose and insulin sensitivity by lowering normal and fasting glucose level and by increasing insulin sensitivity (Khanh V, 2015).The roots of the Coyote Melon also contain dichloromethane (DCM) which has been found to decrease fasting blood glucose levels, increased serum insulin levels and improved oral glucose tolerance (Zhaoxia Liu, 2013).

- **Nopal cactus/prickly pear (Opuntia)** – is a form of cactus native to North and South America. Nopal is one of the mineral-dense foods on the planet. Nopal contains calcium, copper, iron, magnesium, manganese, phosphorous, potassium, selenium, sodium, zinc, all B vitamins except B12, Vitamin A, C, and E. Some other constituents are pectin, fiber and 17 amino acids of which 8 are essential amino acids. Nopal has been used to treat diabetes for a long time in Central America and by the American Indians. Nopal has been shown to significantly decrease blood glucose values in type 2 diabetes patients (Gutierrez, 1998). Another study fed people with type 2 diabetes a high carb breakfast with and without Nopal added. The results found that nopal could reduce glucose, serum insulin, and plasma glucose-dependent insulinotropic peptide (GIP) peaks as well as increase antioxidant activity in people with type 2 diabetes (J, 2014).

- **Nettle /Stinging Nettle (Urtica Dioica) –** is a leafy herbaceous plant that grows as a wild green all over the world. Nettle is one of the most nutrient dense plants in nature. Nettle has 4 times the amount of Vitamin C versus one medium sized orange. Nettle also contains Vitamins A, B1, K, potassium, calcium, silicon, ferric oxide (non-hemoglobin iron). As well as agglutinin, acetophenone, alkaloids, acetylcholine, chlorogenic acid, butyric acid, Terminalia, caffeic acid, carbonic acid, choline, histamine, coumaric acid, formic acid, pantothenic acid, kaempferol, coproporphyrin, lectin, lecithin, ermin, linoleic and linolenic acids, palmitic acid, xanthophyll, quercetin, quinic acid, serotonin, stigmasterol, terpenes, violaxanthin, and succinic acid in its chemical content (1. Ayan AK, 2006). 30% to 40% of Nettle is mainly protein and also high in fiber, which helps regulate blood pressure and digestion. In studies, nettle enhanced insulin sensitivity and insulin-stimulated glucose metabolism in skeletal muscles. The results of those studies show nettle as a beneficial supplement for metabolic disease such as insulin resistance (Diana N. Obanda, 2016).

## Other herbs for Diabetes

- **Afara/Limba/Ofram/Korina (Terminalia superba)** – is a tree that is native to the West Africa area and has been used as a medicinal remedy for centuries. The bark of the tree is often chewed or made into a tea. The bark of the tree contains gallic acid and methyl gallate, which have shown significant ability to lower glucose. Also, alcohol extracts from the bark also showed to be vasorelaxant and antidiabetic activities. One study conducted on rats induced with Diabetes showed that extracts from the Limba tree can reverse hyperglycemia, thus having antidiabetic properties (Kamtchouing P, 2006).

- **Neem (Azadirachta indica)** – is a green tree native to South Asia countries. In Indian mythology, the tree is divine in origin and was formed from drops of nectar from the heavens. Neem is derived from Sanskrit Nimba which translates to bestow health (Puri, 1999). Neem oil has shown the ability to lower glucose and is widely used in India for treatment of diabetes. Diabetes is directly related to the pancreas being compromised and can lead to pancreatic cancer. Neem oil contains nimbolide, in laboratory test nimbolide reduced the capacity of pancreatic cancer cells to multiply and metabolize by 70%, so the cancer cells did not spread.

The cancerous cells seemed attacked from all angles from using nimbolide (Subramani R, 2016).

- **Aloe Vera (Aloe barbadensis miller)** – the earliest recorded human use of aloe vera was found in the Ebers Papyrus (an Egyptian medical scroll) in the 16th (Amar Surjushe, 2008). Its origins are located in Africa going about 6000 years ago but can now be found worldwide. Aloe vera contains Vitamins A, C, E, B12, folic acid, calcium, chromium, copper, selenium, magnesium, manganese, potassium, sodium, zinc, sugars (glucose and fructose), hormones and 20 out of the 22 amino acids and 7 out of 8 essential amino plus other phytonutrients. Aloe vera has shown significant reduction in fasting blood glucose levels and also shown to be able to lower HbA1c (Minh Q Ngo, D, & Sachin A Shah, 2010).

- **Rosemary (Rosmarinus officinalis) and Greek Oregano (Origanum Vulgare) and Mexican Oregano (Lippia Graveolens)** – are herbs that most people know about but few know their medicinal qualities. These herbs contain beneficial phytonutrients and flavonoids. Gallic acid was found in these pair of herbs in a high concentration. Gallic acid has glucose lowering effects on the body and was shown to inhibit enzymes that play a role in insulin secretion and insulin signaling (Allyson M Bower, 2014).

# Chapter 7: Cholesterol

High cholesterol is not a health condition but a sign of underlying health problems that need proper treatment. High cholesterol is not as harmful as you think! Cholesterol is Vital for proper function of the body. Cholesterol is a Greek word "chole" means bile, "stereos" means solid, and the chemical suffix "ol" means alcohol. Cholesterol is an organic chemical substance; classified as a waxy steroid of fat. In 1758 French Dr. Francois Poulletier de la Salle isolated cholesterol. He isolated it from in a solid form from gallstones.

**Proven facts on Cholesterol:**

1. Cholesterol is either bad or unhealthy, it is an essential compound for every cell structure. Cholesterol is a must for the proper functioning of the brain and nerves.

2. Low cholesterol levels are dangerous and may increase the risk towards hemorrhagic stroke and cancer.

3. If somehow you could remove all the cholesterol from the body, the body would disintegrate.

4. The vital organs brain and liver contain a lot of cholesterol.

5. 25% of the total cholesterol in the body is found in the brain.

6. Cholesterol builds and maintains cell membranes.

7. Cholesterol is essential for the cell membranes of the brain and transmission of neurotransmitters.

8. Cellular communication gets impaired without cholesterol, cognition and memory function affected.

9. Cholesterol insulates neurons (a specialized cell transmitting nerve impulses)

10. Cholesterol regulates membrane fluidity over different physiological temperatures

11. Cholesterol does intracellular transportation, cell signals, and nerve conductions

12. The liver uses cholesterol to produce bile and stored in the gallbladder

13. Fat digestion requires bile acid; it dissolves and helps intestinal absorption of fat

14. The liver uses cholesterol to produce fat-soluble vitamins: A, D, E, and K

15. Cholesterol is essential for the synthesis of the steroid hormones, such hormones are the adrenal and sex hormones

16. The adrenal hormones are cortisol and aldosterone

17. The sex hormones are progesterone, estrogen, and testosterone

If cholesterol has numerous vital functions in the body then how can it harm you? High cholesterol may even be protective, except for the case of familial hypercholesterolemia. A high cholesterol level in older people is actually shielding. High cholesterol also called hypercholesterolemia and hyperlipidemia. High cholesterol is a condition characterized by an elevated lipoproteins level.

The dietary cholesterol represents only 1/3 of the body total cholesterol needs. The remaining comes from liver production. Blood is watery and cholesterol is fatty, these two do not mix. So cholesterol needs to carry with a protein cover. This combination of lipid and protein is called lipoproteins. Transportation of cholesterol needs to be carried in small packages lipoproteins (HDL, LDL, VLDL).

- Low-density lipoprotein (LDL) is considered a bad cholesterol. LDL transports cholesterol and triglycerides from the liver to the peripheral tissues

- High-density lipoprotein (HDL) is considered good cholesterol. HDL carries out reverse cholesterol transport and hopes to prevent heart conditions

- Very-low-density lipoprotein (VLDL) also considered a bad cholesterol. VLDL transports cholesterol and triglycerides from the liver to the peripheral tissues

- Triglycerides are present in the blood and stored in the fat cells. They are the primary sources of energy and common fat type present throughout the body

- Total cholesterol is a measurement of the entire cholesterol by breaking down all the lipoproteins.

High cholesterol is not a disease but may be a sign of other health condition like inflammation or infection. Studies show low cholesterol levels may be a sign of undiagnosed cancer. High cholesterol is the sign towards heart attack or stroke risk. Most Doctors treat the symptoms and not the conditions. They try and suppress the high cholesterol level by prescribing cholesterol-lowering medication. Treating the underlying cause of high cholesterol can lower cholesterol without medications. Elevated cholesterol is not from high-fat diet, but from high carbohydrates (sugar is deadly). Changes in lifestyle are the safest way to lower cholesterol. Eating a healthy diet, losing weight and exercise are the 3 fundamental steps to lowering cholesterol.

Scientist first found cholesterol plaque (deposits) in the people who died from heart conditions. They concluded that their deaths were due to high cholesterol levels in the blood. But cholesterol was probably there to help heal some problems such as inflammation. Blaming cholesterol for the cause of heart disease is like blaming a fireman for putting out a fire. Calcium deposits and inflammation are the real culprits that form plaque in the arteries. A deficiency in Vitamin K may be the cause for the calcium deposits in the arteries. High cholesterol risks are due to prolong management of cholesterol along with inflammation.

**Different classifications of the most prescribed hyperlipidemia medications:**

- Statins are the most prescribed medication used to lower cholesterol. The use of statins are recommended for 1) People with previous cardiovascular disease, 2) people with have high LDL cholesterol, 3) individuals between 40 and 75 with diabetes, 4) people who have increased the chance for cardiovascular problems in the next 10 years. You can tell the statins by their pharmaceutical names Lipitor (atorvastatin), Crestor (rosuvastatin), Zocor (simvastatin), Pravachol (pravastatin), Mevacor (lovastatin) and Lescol (fluvastatin). Statins are classified as an HMG- CoA reductase inhibitors. HMG- CoA is an enzyme produced in the liver that is responsible for making cholesterol, Co-Enzyme Q10 and dolichol. These 3 are all inhibited in the body by taking statin medications. Co-Enzyme Q10 is required by every cell in the body to produce energy. The heart and the brain are the 2 most energy dependent organs in the body. Dolichol is a compound in the body that is involved in intracellular activities like message transport, neuropeptide formation and mitochondrial DNA error correction. While statin drugs do lower your cholesterol, they do not lower your risk of heart disease, heart attacks or strokes. Some side effects of Statins are diabetes, cancer, muscle weakness, depression, mental cognition decline, nausea, shortness of breath, ringing in the ears, liver damage, heart failure, Pancreatitis, sexual dysfunction and swelling to name a few.

- **Bile Acid Sequestrant/ Resins (Welchol)** – The liver produces bile, bile salts and bile acids. Once the bile is created most of it travels to the gallbladder where it gets stored and purified until it's needed. Whenever we eat and the food travels down to the Duodenum (upper portion of the small intestines), the gallbladder releases the purified form of bile salts and bile acids into the small intestines to interact with the food. The mixture of food and bile salts and acids travels down to the Ileum (the lower part of the small intestines) and up to 90% gets recycled. The recycled bile salts and acids get circulated via the Enterohepatic Circulation. Since 90 % bile salts and acids are getting recycled, the body doesn't need to make any extra cholesterol. Resins lower the amount of cholesterol in the body by blocking Enterohepatic Circulation. Blocking the enterohepatic circulation means the body can't recycle the bile salts and acids, thus new bile has to be produced and cholesterol is needed in the production of bile. By making new bile cholesterol levels are lowered in the body. Some side effects of resins are gallstones, weight loss, gastrointestinal problems, can inhibit the absorption of fat-soluble vitamins and can increase the rate of colon cancer.

- **Fibrates (Fenofibrate, Gemfibrozil)** – these drugs are used prescribed when there are elevated amounts of triglycerides, fats, or fatty acids in the body. Fibrates increase the production of enzyme LPL (lipoprotein lipase), which breaks down triglycerides and fats in the body. Fibrates also increase the production of ApoC1 and ApoC 2 (Apolipoprotein) which increase the uptake of the breakdown of the fats and helps expel them from the body. Some side effects are gastrointestinal problems rash, fever, anemia, headache and gallstones.

- **Niacin (Niaspan)** – Vitamin B3 also known as niacin is vital for the body to turn carbohydrates into glucose. Niacin works by stopping the release of triglycerides from stored body fat and by blocking the liver from producing more from blood glucose by blocking key enzymes. Thus lowering LDL cholesterol and increasing HDL cholesterol. The daily requirement for

Niacin is 20mg to 35mg a day, prescription niacin to lower cholesterol is 50 times more than the daily requirement. Side effects are flushing (skin turning red), nausea, liver disease, gallbladder disease, glucose intolerance, increased uric acid, ulcers, blurred vision, and a decrease in thyroid function.

The number needed to treat for people who took statins for 5 years: 1 in 104 were helped (prevented heart attack), 1 in 154 were helped (prevented a stroke), none were helped (life saved)

The number needed to harm for people who took statins for 5 years: 1 in 50 were harmed (developed Diabetes), 1 in 10 were harmed (muscle damage)

The benefits in Percentage: 98% so no benefit, 0% were helped (life saved), 0.96% were helped by preventing a heart attack, 0.65% were helped by preventing a Stroke (Melody Ryan, 1999).

## Ayurveda/Rasayana for cholesterol

Way before the western world knew what cholesterol was Ayurveda practitioners understood two primary chemical reactions in the body. The catabolic reaction, which is the breaking down of compounds into smaller ones and releasing heat, governed by Vata Dosha. The anabolic reaction, which is the building up of larger molecules or storing energy, governed by Kapha Dosha. Kapha dosha is heavily involved and influences cholesterol levels in the body. Kapha dosha qualities are heavy, dense, cold, oily, liquid and dull. These qualities beautifully express the fatty like substances in the blood like lipids, lipoprotein, triglycerides, and cholesterol. In Ayurveda, the thyroid function has an enormous impact on the metabolism of the peripheral tissues. A malfunctioning in the thyroid gland (hypothyroidism) leads to decreases in the thyroxine hormones, which results in decrease utilization of the fatty substances like cholesterol from the peripheral tissues. Therefore the increased storage of lipids and fatty substances in the fat tissue and the blood.

## Ayurveda/Rasayana herbs cholesterol

- **Agni/Chitrak (Plumbago zeylanica)** – is a herbaceous plant native to the Pacific and Hawaiian islands but can found in areas of India as well. Chitrak has a bitter ras (taste) and pacifies Kapha and Vata imbalances. One of the main constituents of Chitrak is plumbagin, which was shown to enhance fecal removal of cholesterol and phospholipids (Purushothaman, 1985). As well as the prevention of accumulation of cholesterol and triglycerides in the liver (Sharma I., 1991).

- **Kutki/Katuki (Picrorhiza Kurroa)** - is a plant that grows 3000 feet above sea level in the Himalayans Mountains. In the Sanskrit language the meaning of Kutki is bitter. Kutki is one of the most used herbs in Ayurveda to treat liver imbalances. It helps to increase contractions of the gallbladder and take out secretions, which improves digestion, regulation of fat, proteins and carbohydrate metabolism. Kutki balances Kapha and pitta doshas. Kutki has numerous phytonutrients in its constituents, one phytonutrient is Picroliv. Picroliv was able to lower serum lipids (total, VLDL and LDL cholesterol) (Khanna, Chander, & Kapoor, 1994). Cholesterol biosynthesis in the liver was inhibited and the excretion of bile acids was increased by Picroliv (Tandon, Rastogi, Shukla, Kapoor, & Srimal, 1995).

## TCM Cholesterol

In TCM cholesterol is a recent discovery by westerners, as a result, there is no TCM equivalent specifically for cholesterol. However, there are plenty of herbs used in TCM that indirectly affect cholesterol. The TCM approach is to use herbs to strengthen the stomach and liver, so the cholesterol in the body will be broken down and pushed out more effectively. The stomach which is part of the Yang earth organ meridian is called the "Sea of Nourishment", this is where the food is broken down into its nutritional components. In TCM the stomach is where Chi is extracted from the food. The liver in TCM is part of the Yin wood organ-meridian system and any unbalances in the liver can lead to high cholesterol or other symptoms.

## TCM herbs for Cholesterol

- **Ze Xie/Alisma/Water Plantain tuber (Alisma Plantago- Aquatica)** – is a plant that grows in shallow waters and can be found worldwide. Alisma is sweet in taste and cold which acts on the kidney, liver and gallstones meridians. The plants rhizomes (roots) are used medicinally. Alisma contains Vitamin B-12, biotin, resin, alkaloids, amino acids, essential oils, and other phytonutrients. Two of the phytonutrients are alisol A and alisol B triterpenes. These have shown in human trials to reduce serum triglycerides level as well as cholesterol level. It also increased HDL level and the ratio of HDL to total cholesterol (Wang, 1983).

- **Bupleurum/ Chai Hu (Bupleurum falcatum)** - is a plant native to China that has been used for at least 2000 years. Bupleurum is the most used liver cleansing herb in TCM. Said to disperse Qi (blood) and clear heat from the liver organ meridian. Bupleurum contains a series of triterpenes like saikosaponins and saikogenins. These are known to raise levels of HDL (good cholesterol) and lower levels of LDL (bad cholesterol), also preventing platelets from accumulating in the arteries leading to atherosclerosis. Bupleurum was shown to increase to lower cholesterol by increasing cholesterol excretion in bile (Chang, 1987).

## Electric/Alkaline cholesterol

The liver is the second biggest organ in the body and it plays a key role in overall detoxification of foreign materials from the blood and the body. The liver also houses important nutrients and aids in the assimilation and utilization of nutrients that are extracted from the foods we consume. The liver is where cholesterol is created and distributed throughout the body. The name of the Liver should tell you its importance, without the liver u can't live. The liver is one of the powerfully rejuvenating organs, it's self-regenerating. The body only needs 25% of a functioning liver for it to come back to a holistic state. In general, it takes the liver about 3 ½ years with consistent healthy lifestyle choices to fully heal the liver. Herbs used to treat the liver are recommended to use.

- **Yellow dock/ curly dock (Rumex Crispus) –** has been used by the Native American Indians since ancient times. Yellow dock contains vitamin A, C, calcium, selenium, magnesium, iron, phosphorous and anthraquinones like Emodins. Yellow dock is called a cholagogue because it stimulates the production of bile and digestive fluids. The anthraquinones in yellow dock stimulate the release of bile and different enzymes. As a detox yellow dock helps remove waste in the intestinal tract by stimulating bowel movements, as well as an increase of urination which helps in toxin elimination.

- **Burdock roots/gobo (Arctium lappa)** – is a plant native to North America and China and has been used medicinally for centuries. The roots of the plants are where the major constituent is found. Burdock root contains over 66 different components. One component is inulin which has been shown to be effective for lowering total serum cholesterol and triglycerides in clinical research (Guo, et al., 2012). Inulin is found in the roots of plants and helps the plant to store energy and regulate its internal temperature. As a digestive enzyme inulin attaches to toxins, waste and fat and cholesterol platelets. Inulin lowered LDL by blocking absorption of dietary cholesterol (Moreno Franco B, 2014).

## Other herbs for cholesterol

- **Dandelion roots (Taraxacum officinale)** – is one of the most common herbs that grow all over this world. Used for centuries by indigenous people as a natural detoxifier and blood cleanser. The name Dandelion refers to the French term "dent de lion", meaning lion's tooth. Dandelion roots are classified as "alternatives" which alter the condition of the blood by gathering nutrients and removing metabolic waste. Dandelion contains taraxacin (gives its bitter taste) which promotes the flow of bile and supports digestion. High in pectin fiber, which lowers cholesterol and binds to toxins and expels waste from the body. In a 4-week study, dandelion root showed decreased levels of triglycerides and LDL. Dandelion root also prevented cholesterol from becoming oxidized which promotes inflammation and arterial plaque buildup (Ung-Kyu Choi, 2010).

- **Milk thistle/holy thistle (Silybum marianun)** – is a common weed in California and has been used medicinally throughout ancient times. Milk thistle contains an antioxidant ingredient called silymarin. Silymarin is a compound that protects the liver and supports the detoxification and rejuvenation of the liver organ. Silymarin repairs the exterior layer of liver cells. This process stops toxins from getting in, blocking them and removing them from the body. Milk thistle increased the flow of bile flow and helps in the breakdown of excess fats and cholesterol accumulating in the body and liver. In a double-blind study, silymarin was shown to decrease total cholesterol, LDL, and triglycerides levels (Huseini HF, 2006).

# **Chapter 8: Anticoagulant**

Whole blood contains a liquid portion (plasma) and formed elements (blood cells). Plasma is yellowish in color and is made up of 92% water, metabolic proteins, globulins, clotting factors, hormones, and all other chemicals and gases to support normal body functions. Serum is the liquid portion of the blood after a clot has formed. The blood cells are red which account for about 50% of the blood and white which account for 1% to 2% of all the blood. Red blood cells carry oxygen throughout the body and contain platelets. The white blood cells are the immune cells. The bone marrow is the site of hemopoiesis, which is the production of blood cells and platelets. Any component of the blood is made in the bone marrow like the humerus, radius, ulna, femur, tibia and fibula bones. The marrow is located in the middle of the bones houses stem cells. Stem cells are undifferentiated cells and can become any time of blood cells either red, white or platelets. The blood needs to clot, if not a person could bleed to death. However, you don't want blood to clot too much which could prevent the blood from flowing leading to a stroke or a heart attack. Whenever the human tissue is injured and blood escapes there are a series of reactions that go off in the body. In the blood are platelets (small cell pieces) that start releasing clotting factors whenever injury happens. These clotting factors ignite a series of reactions in the blood.

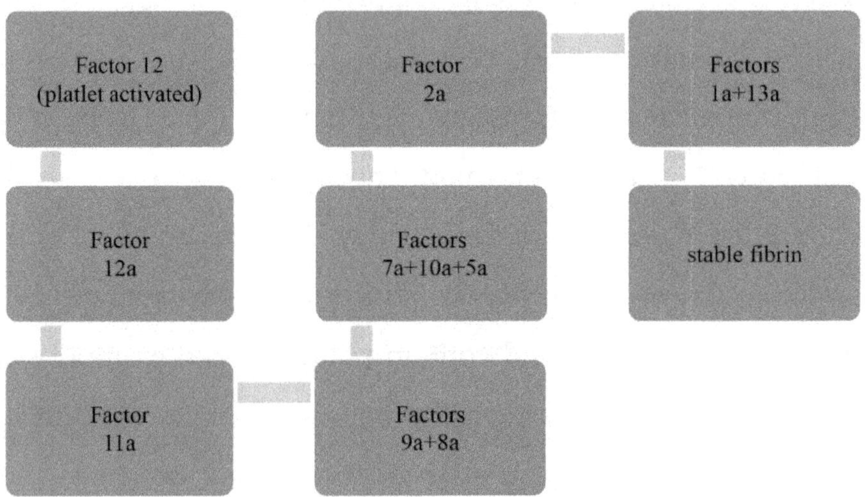


Factors 9a, 10a, 7a, 2a and stabilized fibrin all require calcium to be activated

Factors 9a, 10a, 7a, and 2a all require vitamin K to be produced in the liver in the un-activated form.

Factor 10a is where inactive prothrombin turns into active thrombin (2a)

The active thrombin (2a) activates Fibrinogen (1a)

Fibrinogen (1a) activates stable Fibrin

Prothrombin- 'pro' before thrombin, is a protein that is inactive and changes shape once it receives the signal from the platelets to turn to thrombin (the active version)

Fibrinogen is a protein that is soluble, this means it is dissolved in the blood, is activated by thrombin to turn into Fibrin which is insoluble, which comes out of the blood and forms fiber chains that cause the blood to clot.

**Different classifications of the commonly prescribed prescriptions**

- **Platelet aggregation inhibitors (Aspirin)** - when a platelet becomes activated Arachidonic acid is released from the membranes phospholipids. Then it gets converted to Prostaglandin H2 by cox -1 enzyme. The prostaglandin H2 is converted to Thromboxane A2 which is released from the platelet to stimulate activation of new platelets. Aspirin works by irreversible inactivating cox-1 enzyme thus effectively disrupting clot formation. Common side effects easily bruised, excessive bleeding, jaundice (yellowing of the skin and eyes) and dizziness.

- **Platelet aggregation inhibitors (Plavix)** - activated platelets release chemical mediators, one of them is ADP. ADP binds to the cell receptor P2Y12 leading to the activation of glycoprotein2b3a receptors which are required for fibrin cross-linking to other platelets. Plavix works by blocking P2Y12 cell receptors which inhibits platelet aggregation and thus clot formation. Some side effects are itching, diarrhea, skin redness, jaundice (yellowing of the skin and eyes) and unusual bleeding.

- **Anticoagulants (Heparin)** - these drugs bind to the natural anticoagulants circulating in the blood called Antithrombin. The primary function of antithrombin is to deactivate factor 10a and 2a (thrombin). These drugs bind to antithrombin and accelerate their activity. Some side effects of heparin are bleeding, pain, itching of feet and skin color change.

- **Anticoagulants (Warfarin)** – Vitamin K is responsible for the activation of factors 9,10,7 and 2. These factors are inactive until carboxylated by Vitamin K. The reduced form of Vitamin K initiates the clotting factor. Warfarin inhibits Vitamin K regeneration used in the clotting synthesis. One of the disadvantages of warfarin is that it has a narrow therapeutic window and had has been associated with many drug to drug and drug to food reactions. Some side effects are easily bruised, excessive bleeding, urine different color, joint and stomach pain, and dizziness.

The number needed to treat for a person taking aspirin daily for one year to prevent a first heart attack or stroke: 1 in 1667 cardiovascular problem prevented, none prevented death, and 1 in 2000 prevented non-fatal heart attack and 1 in 10,000 prevented a fatal stroke (Antithrombotic Trialsts' (ATT) Collaboration, 2009).

The number needed to harm for a person taking aspirin daily for one year to prevent a first heart attack or stroke: 1 in 3333 harmed by a major bleeding event. (Antithrombotic Trialsts' (ATT) Collaboration, 2009)

The number needed to treat for a person taking Plavix daily for one year to prevent cardiovascular disease and who have had heart attacks or strokes: 1 in 50 cardiovascular problems prevented, 1 in 77 non- fatal heart attack prevented, 1 in 200 non-fatal strokes prevented, 1 in 333 death prevented (Collaboration, 2002).

The number needed to harm for a person taking Plavix daily for one year to prevent cardiovascular disease and who have had heart attacks or strokes: 1 in 400 had a major bleeding event, 1 in 71 had a rash and 1 in 91 experienced diarrhea (Collaboration, 2002) .

The number needed to treat for a person taking Warfarin daily for 1.5 years for primary stroke prevention (no prior stroke): 1 in 25 prevented stroke, 1 in 42 prevented death from any cause (Aquilar MI, 2005).

The number needed to harm for a person taking Warfarin daily for 1.5 years for primary stroke prevention (no prior stroke): 1 in 25 was harmed (having bleeding) and 1 in 384 was harmed (intracranial hemorrhage) (Aquilar MI, 2005).

The number needed to treat for a person using heparin to reduce the occurrence of myocardial infarction: 1 in 33 prevented myocardial infarction (Magee KD, 2008)

The number needed to harm for the increased incidence of bleeding: 1 in 17 were harmed (having bleeding) (Magee KD, 2008).

## TCM

In TCM the term Blood stagnation refers to the loss of blood functions. In TCM, when there is a blockage there is a pain. The pain associated with blood stagnation is a fixed and stabbing pain. The blood is dark purple in color and contains blood clots. There are two functions of the blood in TCM to nourish the body and the blood is the basic material of the spiritual activity. Some signs of stagnation are mood swings, sleeping problems, emotional problems (phobia). Dry skin and scaly skin are also indicators of blood stagnation since the blood nourishes the body. In TCM the tongue is called the off-shot of the heart because there are a lot of vessels and blood located in the tongue area. If there is blood stagnation there will be dryness in the body causing dry mouth. Also in TCM the stagnation of the blood leads to stagnation of Ying energy which is manifested as phlegm or excessive mucus in the body as well.

## Herb for blood stagnation

- **Dong Quai/Tang Kuei (Angelica Sinensis)** – is a plant related to the celery family that grows in the mountains of China, Korea, and Japan. Dong Quai has been used in TCM for 1000's of years medicinally. Dong Quai contains Vitamins A, C, E, and B12, folate, ferulic acid, calcium, magnesium, carotenoids, essential oils, and other phytonutrients. Dong Quai is one of the few herbs to contain natural coumarins, coumarin inhibits platelet aggregation and thin out the blood naturally. Dong Quai has been used to treat blood stagnation in TCM traditionally. Dong Quai should not be taken if you are currently on any anticoagulant medications.

## Ayurveda/Rasayana herb for blood stagnation

- **Bhringraj/false daisy/Han Lian Cao (Eclipta prostrata)** - is a common plant that grows in wet and muddy conditions. False daisy can be found worldwide and has been used in TCM and Ayurveda medicine for centuries. Traditionally used as a liver and blood tonic. False Daisy main constituent is wedelolactone, which is a complex coumarin. Coumarin is similar to Coumadin and has been shown to reduce platelet formation and increase blood flow. False daisy should not be taken if you are currently on any anticoagulant medications.

## Alkaline/ Electric Herb

- **Guinea Hen Weed/Anumu /Garlic Weed (Petivera Alliacea)** - indigenous to the Amazon rainforest and the tropical areas of the Caribbean, Central and South America and Africa. Anumu grows in warm and tropical climates. Anumu constituents are flavonoids, steroids, sulfur, astilbin, proline, stearic acid and coumarin. Because of the coumarin, Anumu is used as a natural blood thinner. Anumu should not be taken if you are currently on any anticoagulant medications. Women who are pregnant are advised not to take this as well.

## Anticoagulant alternatives

- **Turmeric/Indian Saffron (Curcuma longa)** – is a plant related to the ginger family Zingiberaceae, which is native to South Asia. In Ayurveda turmeric has been used for at least 4000 years medicinally. Over 100 different constituents have been found in turmeric. The two most prevalent are turmerone (a volatile oil) and curcuminoids (coloring agent) (Prasad S, 2011). Turmeric is many overall health benefits in the body. Clinical studies have shown that the curcumin found in turmeric disrupted thrombin activities, thus giving it anticoagulant factors (Kim DC, 2012). Turmeric should not be used if taking any anticoagulant medications.

- **Boldo (Peumus boldus)** – is a plant native to Chile and can be found as far back as the Inca civilization in use. Has been used for thousands of years as a powerful detoxifying herb especially for the liver. Constituents are flavonoids, resin tannins, essential oils camphor, cineole, Linalool, ascaridole, limonene and alkaloids. The herb also contains coumarins, which thin out the blood and inhibit platelet aggregation. Boldo should not be used if taking any anticoagulant medications.

# Chapter 9: anti-inflammatory

Inflammation will occur anytime damage or injury has been afflicted to vascularized tissue. The inflammatory process initially starts off with a vascular response. The inflammatory process is represented by 4 signs: redness (increased circulation and vasodilation in injured tissues in response to chemical messengers), heat (given off by increased blood flow), swelling ( increased fluid escaping into the tissue as blood vessels dilate and prevents spread of infection) and pain (stimulation of nerve endings). When damage occurs the blood vessels in that area will dilate, increasing the amount of blood flow headed to the injured site. The endothelium cells (cells that line the inside of the blood vessel) responded to pro-inflammatory chemical messengers which can tell them to constrict and get smaller, which means that the space between one endothelium cell to the next gets larger. The blood flow that's coming thru those vessels can be pushed out of the blood vessel into the surrounding tissue at the area where it's injured. The vascular/inflammatory response is vasodilation and endothelium constriction, which only occur because of chemical messengers of inflammation that has been released from surrounding cells. Some chemical messengers of inflammation are Prostaglandins, Leukotrienes, Nitric Oxide, Bradykinins, Histamines, and Cytokines.

The cells in the body are surrounded by a phospholipid bilayer. Phospholipids have a phosphate head that is hydrophilic (likes water) and 2 fatty acid lipid tails that are hydrophobic (don't like water). A small portion of the fatty acid tail is called Arachidonic acid. Arachidonic acid produces prostaglandins and leukotrienes.

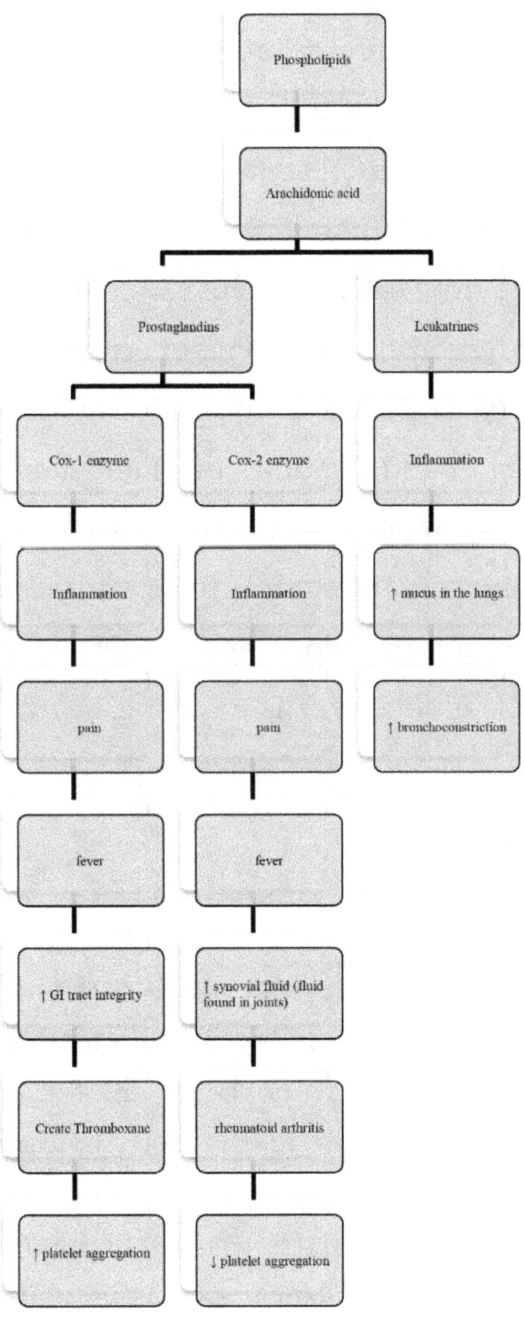
Phospholipids
Arachidonic acid
Prostaglandins
Leukatrines
Cox-1 enzyme
Cox-2 enzyme
Inflammation
Inflammation
Inflammation
↑ mucus in the lungs
pain
pain
↑ bronchoconstriction
fever
fever
↑ GI tract integrity
↑ synovial fluid (fluid found in joints)
Create Thromboxane
rheumatoid arthritis
↑ platelet aggregation
↓ platelet aggregation

A fever is the body normal response anytime there is an infection. Whenever the body senses a foreign material it sends a signal to the hypothalamus to raise the temperature to kill the foreign material. Anything that causes fevers is known as pyrogens; 'pyro=heat". Pyrogens can come from bacteria or be a chemical response to inflammatory chemical messengers. Fevers can be beneficial if it's a low-grade fever. A fever in the body inhibits multiplication of temperature sensitive microorganisms, impedes nutrition of bacteria by reducing the availability of iron, and increase metabolism and stimulates immune reactions and protective physiological process. A low-grade fever is anything below 102 degrees Celsius

## Prescribed drugs for inflammation

- **(NSAIDs) Nonsteroidal Anti-inflammatory Drugs (Aspirin, Ibuprofen, Naproxen) –** these drugs reduce the inflammatory response by inhibiting both cox-1 and cox-2 enzymes in the body. Though both are affected the cox -1 enzyme is slightly more impacted. Often directed to take with food, by inhibiting the cox-1 enzyme these drugs can lower gastrointestinal integrity. In the stomach, there is a mucus lining that protects our stomach from the acid it creates. That acid is Hydrochloric Acid and has a very low pH around 1.5-3. Prostaglandin cox-1 helps us create that mucus lining that protects the stomach. Cox -1 is also responsible for the creation of thromboxane which is responsible for platelet aggregation. By inhibiting that function low dose Aspirin is recommended cardiovascular patients or people prone to strokes and heart attacks to lower platelets in the blood. Some side effects of NSAIDs are stomach pain, gastrointestinal ulcers, liver problems and high blood pressure.

- **(NSAIDs) Nonsteroidal Anti-inflammatory Drugs (Celebrex)** – is a cox- 2 specific inhibitor. Cox -2 prostaglandins are found in high quantities in the synovial fluid. The synovial fluid is found at synovial joints like the knee. If you increase the amount of cox-2 prostaglandins in the synovial fluids by the knee, it will promote inflammation and pain, and can lead to rheumatoid arthritis. By inhibiting cox-2 this drug has been used for arthritis treatment. Cox- 2 is also responsible for lowering platelet aggregation, by inhibiting that function the risk of clotting is increased. One of the major side effects of cox-2 inhibitors are blood clots, increase in the number of platelets in the blood, liver problems and stroke just to name a few.

Arachidonic Acid also creates Leukotriene. Leukotrienes are involved in inflammation, increase mucus secretion in the lungs, and increase bronchoconstriction. All of these are the signs of Asthma. Leukotrienes are involved in the inflammatory process known as asthma. Asthma is a reversible inflammatory disease, inflammation is the root cause of Asthma. Prescription drugs don't stop the production of leukotrienes but bind to the leukotriene cell receptors

- **Leukotriene Reception antagonists (Singular)** – they bind to the leukotriene receptors, thus reducing inflammation, decreasing mucus secretion in the lungs, and opening up the airways. Some side effects of leukotriene reception antagonist are tremors, headache, nausea, fever, sore throat and heartburn.

On top of the kidneys are the adrenal glands. The outer portion of the adrenals is called the cortex and the inner portion is called the medulla. Different hormones/steroids are produced in different layers. In the cortical layer, we produce the steroids cortisol and cortisone, known as Glucocorticoids. These steroids promote the release of glucose (sugar) into the bloodstream. Glucocorticoids role in inflammation is their ability to stop Phospholipids from turning Arachidonic Acid. By that mechanism, they can stop Prostaglandins from being produced and Leukotrienes from being produced. Steroids are lipid base, so they can enter the cell and alter the transcription of genes. The genes they can alter are the pro-inflammatory genes.

- **Synthetic Steroids (Prednisone) -** are a synthetic version of cortisol. Often prescribed for rheumatoid arthritis, inflammation, autoimmune diseases and skin issues to name a few. Some side effects are increased weight gain, low libido, immune malfunction, liver damage, and Diabetes.

These drugs work by inhibiting the inflammatory process. I prefer herbs and lifestyle changes thus getting to the root cause of the inflammation. Inflammation in the body is a key sign that something is wrong. Instead of treating the problem its best to solve it all together. The number needed to treat for NSAIDs are good at inhibiting the inflammatory response. The number needed to treat to reduce the pain over a 4 to 6 hour period for most NSAIDs: 1 in 2 saw a reduction in pain (C.K.S Ong, 2007). The problem with NSAIDs are the long-term effects over time. The number needed to harm for gastrointestinal bleeding with low dose aspirin over a 12 week period once a day was: 1 in 247 were harmed by gastrointestinal bleeding (L, 2006). The number to harm of a person taking Celebrex for osteoarthritis or rheumatoid arthritis for more than 12 weeks once a day were: 1 in 9 were stopped due to lack of efficiency, 1 in 74 were harmed by an adverse event, and 1 in 58 were harmed by a gastrointestinal adverse event (R Andrew Moore, 2006). The number needed to treat for a person taking synthetic steroids for acute COPD (chronic obstructive pulmonary disease) exacerbations were: 1 in 10 were helped and the number needed to harm was 1 in 7 were harmed by adverse drug effects (Walters Jae, 2005).

## TCM inflammation

In TCM pain and inflammation are caused by the stagnation of energy and fluids. When the flow is impeded, pain occurs, signaling to us there is a problem. Pain originates from 3 factors: deficiency (flow of energy/fluids are weak due to deficient Ch'i or blood), obstruction (flow is blocked from injury, swelling, or overeating), and constraint (flow is restricted due to mental and physical constraint). When Ch'i and the blood move unblocked in the body there is no pain. It is essential to keep those moving for optimal health. In TCM a stagnation of Ch'i has a pain that varies in intensity and location, associated with soreness, and occurs with emotional changes. Blood stagnation has a pain that is fixed in location, sharp and stabbing pain, and with swelling. Overall stagnation of Ch'i over time can lead to a condition where the Ch'i can't move the blood and causes it to stagnate or coagulate. This is seen mostly as a case of liver Ch'i stagnation. If the blood becomes deficient, this can cause a loss of Ch'i function, as Ch'i is said to move the blood. Thus a Ch'i deficiency leads to blood stasis.

## TCM herbs for inflammation

- **Zhi Mu (Anemarrhena Rhizoma)** –is a member of the lily family native to China and Japan. Zhi Mu is sweet and bitter in taste and effects the lung, stomach and kidney meridians. Zhi Mu is used to clear heat, purges fire, nourishes Yin and moistens dryness (chief), 2000-06). Zhi Mu has been shown to be a natural cox-2 inhibitor.

- **Huang Bai/Amur Cork Tree (Phellodendron bark)** – is native to Eastern Asia and Northern China and is part of the Rutaceae family. The taste is bitter and cold which affects the liver, kidney, and Bladder meridians. Huang Bai has been used traditionally in TCM to clear heat and dampness, reduce fire, release toxins, eczema, and reduce swollen red, legs and feet. Huang Bai has been shown to have an anti-inflammatory effect by inhibiting cox-2 and other inflammatory chemical messengers (Xian YF, 2011).

## Ayurveda inflammation

The word inflammation signifies "heat" being in the body. Chronic inflammation is too much heat being built up over time. In Ayurveda chronic inflammation is associated with a Pitta dosha (the fire essence) imbalance. Pitta imbalance refers to the red, hot, and tender type of pain and not the swelling caused by fluid retention which is a Kapha dosha imbalance. Fire is associated with the metabolism in Ayurveda. The metabolism digests are food, produces life- generating energy, and burns away waste. The problem lies when the metabolic fire burns too hot, then stagnates or flares up in other areas of the body which cause chronic inflammation. Herbs that help cool the body are used to help chronic inflammation in Ayurveda

## Ayurveda/Rasayana herbs

- **Salai Guggal/Indian Frankincense (Boswellia Serrata) –** is a plant that is native to North Africa and India. Its use in Ayurveda goes back to 700 b.c. in the first recorded medical text Charaka Samhita. Salai Guggal has been used traditionally to treat chronic inflammation on the body. The plant contains many phytonutrients and resins. One of the constituents, in particular, is Boswellic acid, which has been shown as a potent inhibitor of certain enzymes responsible for inflammation (Siddiqui, 2011). In another trial, people with osteoarthritis were treated with Salai Guggal and all patients reported a decrease in knee pain, decrease in swelling of the knee, increase knee flexion and increase in walking distances (Kimmatkar N, 2003).

## Electric/Alkaline Herbs for inflammation

- **Yucca/Spanish dagger (Yucca schidigera) –** is a plant to Mexico and Southwest Regions of America. Traditionally used by Native Americans to treat a number of ailments due to inflammation. Yucca plant has one of the highest constituents of saponins. Saponins are derived from Latin word sapo which means soap, are found naturally in plants and produce soap-like qualities when mixed with water. This lathering effect is good for binding to cholesterol and treating inflammation in the body. Some key saponins in Yucca have been shown to inhibit the enzyme responsible for the production of inducible nitric oxide synthase, which triggers the formation of the inflammatory agent nitric oxide (PR Cheeke, 2006). Resveratrol the chemical associated with the benefits of red wine are found in Yucca as well. In recent studies, resveratrol was shown to inhibit the synthesis and release of pro-inflammatory mediators cox-1 and cox 2 enzymes (Das S, 2007).

## Other herbs for inflammation

- **Pepper Elder/Jointa/Silver Bush (Peperomia Pellucida)** – is an annual plant native to South America and the Caribbean Islands. Pepper Elder has been used by indigenous people for thousands of years to treat numerous ailments including arthritis, gout, and inflammation. As a member of the pepper family, it has a very spicy smell. A liquid extract was tested and showed to interfere with prostaglandin synthesis, thus making it beneficial as an anti-inflammatory alternative (Maria de Fatima Arrigoni-Blank, 2004).

# Chapter 10: Antimicrobial (Antibiotics, Antifungal, Antiviral)

The Prefix 'anti' means against, these types of medications work against microbes (bacteria, fungi, and virus). A newborn baby is born sterile, completely free of microbes. As soon as the baby exits the womb it's exposed to microbes and acquires more over time from family members and environment. The body is a host organism that is home to trillions of microbes. These microbes have a synergistic relationship with the body. There are over 1000 different microbes that make up 1 human being. Majority of the microbes reside in the gastrointestinal tract and are non -pathogenic. Antimicrobial is a common metabolic product of aerobic bacteria (Streptomyces and Bacillus) and fungi (Penicillium and Cephalosporium). Bacteria that produce antimicrobials in the bodywork by releasing chemicals that kill other organisms that inhabit their space. Antimicrobials are those chemicals that are released and occur naturally. Antimicrobial medications are drugs that kill or inhibit microbe cells. There are different types of antimicrobial drugs that affect different parts of the microbe cell and human cell. The most prescribed antibiotics are cell wall inhibitors (Penicillins, Amoxicillin, Cephalexin). These drugs work by attacking the cell wall. Human cells don't have a cell wall, rather a cell membrane. Human cells don't have the 70s ribosome, which drugs like (Clindamycin, Erythromycin) work by attacking. Drugs like Polymyxin affect the cell membranes, which both microbes and human cells have. Ciprofloxacin and Rifampin affects DNA and RNA, which both microbes and human cells have. Drugs like Bactrim which is an antifungal medication affects metabolic pathways and products which effects microbes and human cells.

## Bacteria

Bacteria have many beneficial roles to humans and the ecosystem. In relationship to human cells, bacteria outnumber them 10 to 1. Bacteria aid in digestion, produce vitamins, eliminate toxins, keep harmful bacteria under control, aids in the production of antibodies to harmful bacteria and plays a major overall role in general health. Bacteria are Prokaryotic organisms, which means that they don't have their DNA in a single cell like a nucleus. Majority of the bacteria aren't harmful to humans, the harmful ones are called pathogens.

Pathogenic bacteria make people sick by excreting a toxin. The toxin could be an Exotoxin, which is a toxin excreted outside the cell or an Endotoxin, which is a protein found outside the cell membrane. Most bacteria have cells walls made up of peptidoglycan. Cell wall inhibitors block the synthesis of peptidoglycan. The blockage causes the cell walls to lyse (destruct). These cell wall inhibitors are more effective on young and new growing bacterial cells. The problem with antibiotics isn't their effectiveness, it's the overuse that's the problem. Antibiotics are often prescribed for colds, flu, bronchitis and sore throats which are caused by viruses which antibiotics can't kill. According to the CDC, each year in the United States 47 million unnecessary antibiotic prescriptions are written (Antibiotics Aren't Always the Answer, 2016). The overuse of antibiotics leads to some bacteria becoming resistant. The more potent you try to kill a living substance only the stronger ones will survive and thrive. In the U.S.A, at least 2 million people will become infected with bacteria that are resistant to antibiotics and at least 23,000 will die (Antibiotic/Antimicrobial Resistance, 2017). A type of bacteria resistant to antibiotics would be salmonella. The majority of the antibiotics used in this country are for livestock. In 2015 alone over 34.3 million pounds of antibiotics were used for livestock compared to 7.7 million pounds for human use (Mckenna, 2017). Most of the bacteria in all animals are found in the intestines. The overuse of antibiotics kills some bacteria, but the resistant bacteria survive and thrive.

The importance of bacteria to health has recently become more known. If antibiotics kill bacteria, then probiotics promote bacteria. 80 % of the immune system resides in the gastrointestinal tract, where the majority of the bacteria in the body is found. On average 2 to 3 pounds of total body weight is bacteria. The beneficial bacteria aids in digestion keeps out pathogens and regulates the yeast/fungus in the body. It's important to keep the balance between bacteria for optimal health.

## Fungi/yeast

The human body has a diverse population of fungi, bacteria and viruses when healthy and when diseased. There are over 1.5 million different fungi found on this planet, but only about 300 are known to be pathogenic to humans (Types of Fungal Diseases, 2017). Unlike bacteria, fungi can be found all over the body. Fungi have eukaryotic cells, which mean they have a cell membrane like human cells do. Anyone can get a fungal infection even healthy people. Fungi are common to the environment, and we breathe or come in contact with fungus spores all the time without getting sick. In a person with a weak immune system, the same fungi spores are more likely to cause an infection. Two different fungi are found in abundance in the human body and both are dimorphic fungi, which means they can exist both as a yeast and a fungus in the body. The majority of the skin is colonized by Malassezia fungi, which comes from the family corn smut, a fungus that brings devastation to corn farmers. There are 14 different species of Malassezia fungi, which 8 are associated with humans, and 4 being commonly found (Hort W, 2011). Malassezia initiates inflammatory reactions that have been associated with numerous ailments including dermatitis, dandruff, eczema, and folliculitis by (Charles W. Saunders, 2012). When the immune system has been weakened Malassezia can lead to systematic infections, which are infections that affect the whole body like a cold, Chlamydia, Syphilis, and HIV. Since Malassezia is part of the natural skin flora now, the immune system is constantly exposed to the fungi. Malassezia is found on the skin of healthy people as well. The problem lies when the fungi breach the skin barrier, by way of producing increased amounts of irritating fatty acids that lower the immune system.

The other fungi/yeast found in abundance in the human body is Candida. Over 20 different species of Candida are known pathogen to humans, with Candida albicans being the most common (Fungal Diseases:Candidiasis, 2015). Candida yeast is generally found in the gastrointestinal tract in the body and also reside on the skin and mucus membranes without infection. When an overgrowth happens the condition is called Candidiasis, which is a systematic infection. Candidiasis in the mouth or throat area = thrush (redness or soreness, difficulty swallowing, and cracking at the corners of the mouth), candidiasis in the vaginal area= yeast infection (itching, burning and vaginal discharge), candidiasis in the genital area= yeast infection (itchy rash on the penis) and candida can enter the bloodstream and spread throughout the body. Once in the bloodstream it's called Invasive candidiasis, which is a serious infection that can affect the blood, heart, brain, eyes, bones and other parts of the body (Invasive Candiasis, 2015). Majority of the incidences of Invasive candidiasis occurs in hospitals. According to recent research, at least 70% of all people are affected by Candidiasis ("Biologosts ID Defense Mechanism of Leading Fungal Pathogen"). Candida and other fungi are part of the natural flora of the human body when healthy when the immune system is weakened an overgrowth can happen. Just like bacteria, certain fungi are becoming resistant to prescription antimicrobial medications from there overuse. One study concluded that antibiotic prescriptions may contribute to resistance by reducing bacteria in the gut and create favorable conditions for Candida growth (Ben-Ami R, 2012). According to CDC reports 7% of all Candida isolated in the blood that was tested were resistant to Fluconazole, most were Candida glabrata (Lockhart SR, 2012). Fluconazole is a first line defense antifungal medication and is commonly prescribed. The second line of defense is called echinocandin, which know are becoming more resistant to Candida glabrata, which has already shown resistance to Fluconazole (Vallabhaneni S, 2015). Fungal infections are common among people with a weak immune system. Certain medications have side effects that can lower the immune system and increase the chance of a fungal infection. Corticosteroids (Prednisone, Triamcinolone, Hydrocortisone, Medrol), inhaled corticosteroids (Fluticasone, Budesonide) and tumor necrosis factor inhibitors (Humira, Enbrel) are types of medications that raise the chance of getting a fungal infection (Ali T, 2013). These can cause oral candidiasis (thrush) especially inhaled corticosteroids, invasive Candida infection, histoplasmosis, pneumocystis pneumonia and invasive aspergillosis (Medications that weken Your immune system and fungal infections, 2017).

## Common Side Effects of Antifungal Prescriptions

- Nausea, vomiting

- Itching, hives

- Difficulty Breathing

- Swelling of lips, tongue and face

- Blistering, redness, or skin irritation

## Viruses

Not all viruses are bad, viruses can be found in the gastrointestinal tract, the skin and in the blood. Every person has a unique collection of viruses but some are common among us all. Majority of the viruses found in the body are bacteriophages, which are viruses that target bacteria but can also be found in human cells too. One bacteriophage CrAssphage, which targets bacteria in the gut was found in over 50% of the population. 8% of the entire human genome comes from endogenous retroviruses, which are viruses that entered the genome and over time became a stable part of the inherited genetic material (M.Markovitz, 2014). One human endogenous retrovirus (HERV) was termed HERV-W was detected in placenta cells, indicating that they may play a role during pregnancy and placenta formation (Jean-Luc Blond, 2000). Both bacteria and phages are associated with mucus. In vitro studies have demonstrated that an increase in phage abundance is mucus dependent and protects the mucus from bacterial infection. The relationship is symbiotic between human host and phage that provide an antimicrobial defense that actively protects the mucosal areas (Barr, 2013). With the overuse of Antiviral medication some viruses are becoming more resistant to prescribed medications. Antiviral drug resistance is especially of importance to people with a compromised immune system, where continues viral replication and extended drug exposure lead to the selection of resistant strains. All the medications used for the herpes virus infection target the virus DNA, which human cells have too. The most common are Acyclovir, Valacyclovir and

Famciclovir, which are the first line defense antiviral drugs. One study showed that Acyclovir resistance was as high as 7 % of patients whose immune system was low compared to 0.27% of people whose immune system were non – compromised (Stanska R, 2005). Influenza which is a Flu virus can replicate and change its genetic makeup, which can lead to the virus becoming resistant to one or more of the antiviral prescription drugs used to treat influenza. With HIV medications drug resistance is caused by changes in the virus's genetic structure. HIV has a fast replicating rate and relies on enzymes to replicate inside a human cell. Because of its rapid rate, most mutations are harmless, but some mutations can block drugs from working against the HIV enzymes.

## Some common side effects of Antiviral

- Anemia
- Nausea
- Diaherra
- Headaches
- Vomiting, dizziness

- Insomnia

- Rash

- Numbness, tingling sensation

## TCM antimicrobial

In TCM the early herbal practitioner's came to the understanding that infectious disease progressed differently than damage from the cold. The name wen bing (warm disease) was termed for infectious diseases. The wen bing attacks the exterior of the body and then progresses into the interior. The cause of wen bing has no sound nor smell, and no shape nor shadow (Chen, 2009). Wen bing is transmitted from one person to another by heaven (air) and earth (physical contact) and affects people with low immunity (Xing, 1642). In TCM many bitter and cold herbs are used to treat wen bing.

## TCM Antimicrobial herb

- **Ban Lan Gen/ Woad (Radix isatidis)** – has been used in TCM to treat excess heat in the body for thousands of years. It's very cooling in nature and bitter in taste. Often the plants rhizome (roots) are used medicinally. Ban Lan Gen affects the stomach, heart, lung and liver meridians. Ban Lan Gen has shown antibacterial and antiviral effects, as well as improvement of immune functions and detoxification. One constituent in Ban Len Gen is Indirubin, which was shown to kill human leukemia cells and inhibit virus replication (Hsuan SL, 2009). Extracts of Ban Lan Gen showed potent antiviral activity against human seasonal influenza virus H1N1 and H3N2 (Li Z, 2017). Ban Lan Gen has also shown anti-endotoxin capabilities. An endotoxin is the toxin present inside of a bacterial cell that is released when the cell dies.

- **Astragalus Radix (Astragalus membranaceus)** - one of the most used herbs in TCM. Astragalus is sweet in flavor and affects the spleen, Lung and Triple warmer meridians. In animal studies, astragulus was shown to resist highly infectious viruses and produced high quantities of Interferon. Interferon is a crucial cellular protein that decreases tumor growth and assumed to be effective against cancers caused by viruses. With its immune strengthening abilities, astralagus is being researched for treatment of AIDS. Astralagus was shown to reduce T- suppressor cells, which inhibit the immune system, are found in high numbers in AIDS patients (Teeguarden, 1985).

## Ayurveda/ Rasayana Antimicrobial herb

- **Haritaki (Terminalia chebula)** – is a medium-sized tree that grows in the Himalayan forests in India. Called Airytha –cures all, Vijaya – conquer of diseases, Divya –divine in nature and Bhisak priya – loved by physicians (Puri, Rasayana: Ayurvedic herbs for longevity and rejuvenation, 2003). Over 30% of the dry weight of Haritaki contain tannins, especially gallic acid. Gallic acid is known to be antiviral and antibiotic in its effect on the body. Gallic acid showed cytotoxicity against infected cells while not affecting non-infected cells. Haritaki in clinical trials was shown to be a potent antibacterial against Salmonella (Rani P, 2004), which is resistant to most antibiotics. As an antifungal alternative Harltaki was shown to be effective at reducing the growth of 3 different Candida yeast species (Vonshak, 2003).

## Electric/ Alkaline Antimicrobial herbs

- **Elderberry (Sambucus nigra)** – is a plant that grows in subtropical climates and can be found in North Africa, North America, Asia and Europe. The uses of elderberry are well known in treatment for colds, flu, influenza, and immune increasing abilities. Elderberry contains a high amount of Vitamin C which is a very powerful antioxidant. A toxin or infection in the body is a result of oxidative stress or lack of electrons. Vitamin C is an antioxidant that donates electrons. Elderberry fruit extracts were shown to increase the inducing activity of L. acidophilus (gram-positive bacteria) in dendritic cells, suggesting that they may exert antiviral and immune-enhancing activity (Frøkiær H, 2012). Elderberry was shown to be effective in vitro against 10 strains of influenza viruses, as well elderberry is beneficial to the immune system activation and in the inflammatory process in healthy individuals or in patients with various diseases. Elderberry showed to have an immune protective or immune stimulatory effect when administered to cancer or AIDS patients, in conjunction with chemotherapeutic or other treatments (Barak V, 2001).

- **Sea Moss/ Irish moss (Chondrus crispus) -** like bladderwrack is a seaweed that's found in ocean coastal regions. Sea moss contains essentially all the fundamental building blocks of life. The antimicrobial effects of sea moss were tested on Salmonella, which is an antibiotic-resistant bacteria. Sea Moss water extracts significantly impaired the ability of Salmonella to colonize the digestive tract by enhancing the expression of immune responsive genes (Kulshreshtha

G, 2016). The use of seaweeds also has been tested for its ability to inhibit certain yeast strains. Sea Moss was shown to inhibit and metabolize the sugars in the yeast of Candida species and others (Kostas ET, 2016). Alcohol extracts of sea moss showed antioxidant functions in the body as well as inducing cell apoptosis in damaged cells.

# Chapter 11: Cancer

Is there a link between Cancer and Candida? Recent studies are starting to correlate an association between the two. Candida albicans have been associated with the cancerous process via its opportunistic pathogenic route that takes advantage of people with low immunity, especially those who have had chemotherapy. The most recent research "demonstrates that Candida albicans are capable of promoting cancer by several mechanisms: production of carcinogenic byproducts, triggering inflammation, induction of Th17 response and molecular mimicry. We underline the need not only to control this type of infection during cancer treatment, especially given the major role of this yeast species in nosocomial infections but also find new therapeutic approaches to avoid tumor effect on this fungal species" (Ramirez-Garcia A, 2016). Candida can produce nitrosamines and acetaldehyde, which are carcinogenic to humans. Nitrosamines are cancer-causing molecules produced by nitrates. If the body is short of vitamin C, then nitrosamines are generated from nitrite in the acid environment of the stomach. Long-term consumption of foods containing nitrosamines; cured meats, beer; some cheeses, nonfat dry milk, pickles, salted fish, bacon, or leftover food with high nitrite content, may induce gastrointestinal tumors (Qi-min Zhan1, 2012). Acetaldehyde is a carcinogenic byproduct from drinking alcohol (ethanol). The liver is the main organ where alcohol metabolism takes place, but a small amount also takes place in the pancreas, brain, and gastrointestinal tract. Chronic inflammation in the body can cause damage to tissue and produce chemicals that are normally used for tissue regeneration but misguided when inflammation is chronic. Candida albicans promotes an inflammatory response in the body when an overgrowth happens due to low immunity and chemical exposure. Underlying chronic inflammation can promote tumor cell adhesion. Cell adhesion molecules play a significant role in cancer progression and metastasis. Interactions of cancer cells with endothelium determine the metastatic spread. In addition, direct tumor cell interactions with platelets, leukocytes, and soluble components significantly contribute to cancer cell adhesion, extravasation, and the establishment of metastatic lesions (Gerd Bendas, 2012). In the presence of Candida albicans the body responses by increasing T cells to help fight the fungi, in particular, TH17 cells. TH17 cells promote the inflammatory response

Interleukin factor 17. Interleukin (IL)-17 is the founding member of a novel family of inflammatory cytokines. While the pro-inflammatory properties of IL-17 are key to its host-protective capacity, unrestrained IL-17 signaling is associated with immunopathology, autoimmune disease, and cancer progression (Nilesh Amatya, 2017). TH17 cells enhancement of tumor growth by IL-17 involves direct effects on tumor cells and tumor-associated stromal cells, which have IL-17 receptors on them. A lot of cancers have been associated with an increased level of IL-17 found in the body. Molecular mimicry happens when a foreign antigen shares sequence or structural similarities with self-antigens. Molecular mimicry has typically been characterized by an antibody or T cell level. A protein located on the surface of Candida albicans has similar structural receptor qualities with white blood cells. This mimicry can cause antibodies to be produced against the immune cells that in turn disrupt the anti-tumor and anti-fungal defense of the body.

## Similarities between Fungi and Cancer

1. Both can metabolize nutrients in the absence of oxygen (Moore-Landecker, 1996) (Warburg O, 1930)

2. Both must have sugar in order to thrive (Moore-Landecker, 1996) (Warburg O, 1930)

3. Both die in the absence of sugar (Moore-Landecker, 1996) (Shim, 1998)

4. Both produce corrosive lactic acid (Hiroaki Shime, 2008)

5. Both respond to antifungal medications (Treatment of Fungal Infections Led to Leukemia Remission, 1999) (Mann, 1997)

Cancer cells are the body's own cells that are growing out of control. Cells are in 2 different phases in the body. Interphase (cell growth and DNA replication) and mitosis (cells are dividing, making new cells). The majority of the cells in the body are in interphase while some cells like the hair follicle cells, bone marrow cells and digestive tract cells are more frequent in mitosis. Cancer cells are frequently in mitosis, which enables them to divide more often and turn into tumors. Tumors are a mass collection of cancerous cells. Tumors can form blood vessels to survive in the body. Those blood vessels provide oxygen and nutrients to the tumor which causes the tumor to grow, this process is termed angiogenesis. Cancer cells can be spread to other areas in the body via the blood vessels created by the tumor. The spreading of cancer cells from one area to another is termed metastasis. Chemotherapy and radiation work by targeting the cells that are in mitosis, this is why hair loss is often a byproduct of these two. Also, other cells might be affected as well by the treatment. Cancer and chemotherapy can damage the body's immune system by decreasing the number of white blood cells that fight infection.

## TCM Cancer

In TCM health and disease relate to the balance between Ying and Yang. The body is seen as one, in which the organs, tissues, and other parts have unique functions but operate independently. In this philosophy, health and disease are related to a balance or imbalance of each unique function. The Ch'i meridians which flow throughout the body nourishes each organ-meridian system. If there is a blockage of Ch'i in a certain area the person will become ill. Cancer is usually expressed as inflammation and blood stagnation in the body.

## TCM herbs for Cancer

- **Astragali Radix (Astragalus membranaceus)** – Astragalus is one the more popular herbs used in TCM. Native to China, Mongolia, and Korea it is related to the pea plant family. The rhizome (roots) are harvested after 4 years and used medicinally. Astragalus is an adaptogen, which means it either removes heat or initiates heat depending on the body needs. Astragalus is great for raising the immune system. In a publication of the American Cancer Society, liquid extracts of Astragalus restored the immune functions in 90% of cancer patients studied. That same report of 572 total cancer patients astragalus was shown to promote adrenal cortical function, which is lowered in cancer patients with low immunity. Astragalus also lessened the effects of gastrointestinal toxicity caused by chemotherapy and radiation (Teeguarden, 1985)

- **Poria/ Fu Ling/ China Root (Poria cocos)** – is a mushroom-like fungi that grow on the outside of certain pine trees native to China. The benefits of Poria have been known in eastern culture for thousands of years. Poria is mildly sweet in taste and affects the spleen, lung, kidney, Triple warmer, Bladder, heart, and gallstone meridians. Poria main constituents are triterpenes and polysaccharides. In clinical trials, triterpenes from Poria demonstrate anticancer and anti-invasive effects on human pancreatic cancer cells and can be considered as new therapeutic agents in the treatment of pancreatic cancer (Shujie Cheng, 2013). One polysaccharide of Poria, β-glucan PCM3-II was tested in vitro against breast cancer cells MCF-7. The study showed that PCM3-II reduced proliferation and viability of the MCF-7 cells dose-dependently so that the cancer-cell growth was decreased by 50% (Mei Zhang, 2006). Poria can be combined with Astralagus, this combination is good for people with low immunity and those trying to recover from illness.

## Ayurveda/Rasayana Cancer

In Ayurvedic cancer is diagnosed as inflammatory or non-inflammatory swelling and mentioned either as Granthi (benign tumors) or Arbuda (cancerous tumors). The nervous system (Vata or air), the venous system (Pitta or fire) and the arterial system (Kapha or water) are three basics of Ayurveda and very important for normal body function. In malignant tumors all three systems get out of balance (Tridoshas) and lose mutual synchronicity that causes tissue damage, resulting in critical condition. Tridoshas cause excessive metabolic turmoil resulting in multiplying or increasing number of cancer cells in the body (Roopesh Jain, 2010). Essentially, cancer affects three doshas of the body.

## Ayurveda/ Rasayana herbs for Cancer

- **Gotu Kola (Centella Asiatica)** – is a plant that grows in wetlands and marshy areas and is native to India, Australia and Asia. The main constituents are saponins and triterpenoids. Gotu Kola has shown useful in preventing radiation-induced changes during clinical radiotherapy. Overall body weight loss of the animals in the drug-treated group was significantly less in comparison with the animals that were given radiation only (Kashmira J. Gohil, 2010). Gotu Kola also induced apoptosis (cell death) in different cancer cells. The cancer cells most sensitive to cell line in vitro were MCF-7 breast cancer cells (Babykutty S, 2008). The juice of Gotu Kola plants were shown not to be toxic to normal cells, but reduced liver tumor cells. Thus, it has the potential to be used as a chemopreventive agent to prevent and treat liver cancer (Faridah Hussin, 2014). Gotu Kola contains Asiatic Acid which significantly reduces lung cancer cell growth both in vitro and in vivo and that the associated apoptosis is mediated through mitochondrial damage (Wu T, 2017). Asiatic Acid is being tested for its effectiveness against ovarian cancer and colon cancer as well. In clinical testing on animals, Gotu Kola increased the number of white blood cells, and thus the potential to enhance innate immunity (Maneewan C, 2014).

- **Amla/Amlaki/Indian Gooseberry (Emblica Officinalis) –** is a fruit that is native to India and has many beneficial uses. In taste, amla is one of the few fruits that exhibit 5 out of the 6 different ras and is balanced with all 3 doshas. Amla has the highest amount of Vitamin C found in any other fruit. Vitamin C is a powerful antioxidant, which helps the body get rid of free radicals that can lead to disease and cancer. Amla in research has shown to be cytotoxic to various cancer cells while not affecting the normal cell. Studies have shown that Amla possesses antipyretic, analgesic, adaptogen, cardiovascular protection, gastrointestinal protection, anti-anemia, anti-hypercholesterolemia, antidiarrheal, anti-atherosclerotic, hepatoprotective, nephroprotective, and neuroprotective properties. In addition, experimental studies have shown that Amla and some of its phytochemicals such as gallic acid, ellagic acid, pyrogallol, some norsesquiterpenoids, corilagin, geraniin, elaeocarpusin, and prodelphinidins B1 and B2 also possess antineoplastic effects. Amla is also reported to possess radiomodulatory, chemomodulatory, chemopreventive effects, free radical scavenging, antioxidant, anti-inflammatory, anti-mutagenic and immunomodulatory activities, properties that are efficacious in the treatment and prevention of cancer (Baliga MS, 2011). Amla extract has been demonstrated to have striking anticancer activity against currently incurable cancer using xenograft models. Xenografts are a tissue graft or organ transplant from a donor of a different species from the recipient. Pyrogallol inhibits the growth of lung cancer cells xenografts. Gallo tannin has shown significant tumor response against triple-negative breast cancers and cholangiocarcinoma (cancer that forms in the bile duct). Xenograft models of pancreatic and triple-negative breast cancers showed considerable response to ellagic acid. Recent evidence also indicates ellagic acid may act as a prophylactic, protecting against the onset of prostate or breast cancer in animal models. Gallic acid shows antitumor qualities against lung and osteosarcoma (bone cancer) (Tiejun Zhao, 2015).

## Electric/Alkaline

- **Soursop/Graviola (Annona muricata)** – is a fruit that grows in tropical climates and is native to Central and South America. All parts of the plants are used including, seeds and leaves. Although all parts are beneficial the leaves of the plant stand out for its medicinal properties.

| Plant Part | Area of Study | Effect | Source |
| --- | --- | --- | --- |
| Alcohol extract of the leaves | Lung A549 cancer cells | Mitochondrial-mediated apoptosis, cell cycle arrest at G1 phase | (Hansra DM, 2014) |
| Alcohol extract of the leaves | Colon HT-29 and HCT-116 cancer cells | Mitochondrial-mediated apoptosis, cell cycle arrest G1 phase, suppression of migration and invasion | (Moghadamtousi SZ, 2015) |
| Water extract of the leaves | Rat's prostate | Reduction of prostate size | (N'gouemo P, 1997) |
| Alcohol extract | Breast tissue of mice | Prevention of DMBA- | (Adeyemi DO K. O., 2009) |

| | | | |
|---|---|---|---|
| of the leaves | | induced DNA damage | |
| Alcohol extract of the leaves | Induced skin cancer in mice | Suppression of tumor initiation and promotion | (Adeyemi DO K. O., 2008;2015) |
| Alcohol extract of the leaves | DMH induced colon cancer | Reduction of ACF formation | (Florence NT, 2014) |
| Alcohol extract of the leaves | K562 chronic myeloid leukemia cells | Induction of apoptosis | (Elisya Y, 2014) |
| Leaves boiled in water | Metastatic breast cancer | Stabilization of disease | (Adeyemi DO, 2008) |
| Alcohol extract of the leaves | Induced colon cancer | Reduction of ACF formation | (Ahalya B, 2014) |
| Alcohol extract of the leaves | Colon HT-29 cancer cells | Bioassay-guided isolation of annomuricin E and its apoptosis-inducing effect | (Ahalya B, 2014) |

*(Ms. Sejal Patel, 2016)*

- **Anamu/ Guinea Hen weed/ Garlic weed/ Gully root (Petivera alliacea)** -indigenous to the Amazon rainforest and the tropical areas of the Caribbean, Central and South America and Africa. Anumu grows in warm and tropical climates. In Jamaica, a survey was administered to 100 patients attending the oncology and urology clinics at the University Hospital of the West Indies in Kingston, Jamaica. Over 80% of interviewed patients, engaged medicinal plants in their treatment regimes. Annona muricata (soursop) and Petiveria alliacea (Anamu) were the most commonly used plants for treating breast and prostate cancers, respectively (Foster K, 2017). One of the constituents in Anamu is dibenzyl trisulfide (DTS), which showed anti-proliferative effects in small lung, pancreatic, breast, and prostate cancer cells. Research has identified DTS as a highly selective and isoform-specific RSK1 kinase inhibitor with broad cancer therapeutic potential (Lowe HI, 2014). Anamu should not be used if pregnant or taking blood thinner medications. Anamu is often combined with soursop in Jamaica as a potent anticancer liquid.

## Other herbs for Cancer

- **Black seed oil (Nigella sativa)** - is a native flowering plant native to the southern parts of Asia. In laboratory studies, black seed oil possesses anti-inflammatory, analgesic, anti-diabetic, anti-hyperlipidemic, anti-convulsant, anti-microbial, anti-ulcer, anti-hypertensive, anti-asthmatic and anti-cancer activities. Black seed oil contains many chemical components, but thymoquinone is the most abundant (Dajani EZ, 2016). Treatment with thymoquinone showed significant attenuation of tumorigenic signaling and several other pro-mitogenic, angiogenic, and metastatic factors, with a consequent dose-dependent inhibition of cancer cell growth, migration, and invasion (A.G.M. Mostofa, 2017). Thymoquinone treatment also showed promising results in resistant human breast cancer cells as well as acute lymphoblastic leukemia, melanoma, colon cancer, and cervical cancer. Studies have observed synergistic cytotoxic and other anti-tumorigenic effects of TQ against cancer cells with simultaneous protection of non-cancerous cells from chemotherapy-induced hazardous effects (A.G.M. Mostofa, 2017).

# Resources

158

To learn more about Dr.Sebi and his products:
https://drsebiscellfood.com

One of my personal favorite site for electric herbs:
https://www.purplemossparadise.com

For TCM herbs: https://www.fourseasonsherbs.com

Ayurveda herbs: https://www.ayurvedicherbsdirect.com

# Notes

(n.d.). "Biologists ID Defense Mechanism of Leading Fungal Pathogen". EurekAlert!

1. Ayan AK, C. O. (2006). Ekonomik Önemi ve Tarımı OMÜ. Agricultural faculty, 21(3):357-363.

A.G.M. Mostofa, M. K. (2017). Thymoquinone as a Potential Adjuvant Therapy for Cancer Treatment: Evidence from Preclinical Studies. Front Pharmaco, 8: 295.

Adeyemi DO, K. O. (2008). Effects of Annona muricata (linn) on the morphology of pancreatic islet cells of experimentally induced diabetic wistar rats. Internet J Altern MED, 5:2.

Adeyemi DO, K. O. (2008;2015). Antihyperlipidemic activities of Annona muricata(linn). Internet J Altern Med; Int J Mol Sci, 16:15656.

Adeyemi DO, K. O. (2009). Antihyperglycemic activities of Annona muricata (linn). Afr J Tradit Complement Altern Med, 6:62-69.

Ahalya B, S. K. (2014). Exploration of anti-hyperglycemic and hypolipidemic activities of ethanolic extract of

Annona mucricata bark in alloxan-induced diabetic rats. Int J Pharm Sci Rev Res, 25:21-27.

Ali T, K. S. (2013). Clinical use of anti-TNF therapy and increased risk of infections. Drug, healthcare, and patient safety, 5:79-99.

Allyson M Bower, L. M. (2014). Bioactive Compounds from Culinary Herbs Inhibit a Molecular Target for Type 2 Diabetes Management, Dipeptidyl Peptidase 4. Journal of Agricultural and Food Chemistry, vol 60 issue 26 6147-6158.

Amar Surjushe, R. V. (2008). Aloe vera: A short review. Indian Journal of Dermatology, 53(4): 163-166.

Aniys, A. (2016). Alkaline Herbal Medicine. Lexington: CreateSpace.

Antibiotic/Antimicrobial Resistance. (2017, August 18). Retrieved from Centers for Disease Control and Prevention: www.dcd.com

Antibiotics Aren't Always the Answer. (2016, November 14). Retrieved from Centers for Disease and Prevention: www.cdc.gov

Antithrombotic Trialists' (ATT) Collaboration, B. C. (2009). Asprin in the primary and secondary prevention of vascular disease: a collaborative meta-analysis of individual participant data from randomised trials. Lancet, 373(9678):1849-60.

Aquilar MI, H. R. (2005). Oral anticoagulants for preventing stroke in patients with non- valvular atrial fibrillation and no previous history of stroke or transient ischemic attacks. Cochrane Database Syst Rev, 20(3):cd001927.

Babykutty S, P. J. (2008). Apoptosis induction of Centella asiatica on human breast cancer cells. Afr J Tradit Complement Altern Med, 6(1):9-16.

Baliga MS, D. J. (2011). Amla (Emblica Officinalis Gaertn), a wonder berry in the treatment and prevention of cancer. Eur J Cancer Prev, 20(3):225-39.

Barak V, H. T. (2001). The effect of Sambucol, a black elderberry-based, natural product, on the production of human cytokines: I. Inflammatory cytokines. Eur Cytokine Netw, 12(2):290-6.

Barr, J. J. (2013). Bacteriophage adhering to mucus provide a non-host derived immunity. PNAS, 110(26):10771-10776.

Ben-Ami R, O.-P. K. (2012). Antibiotic exposure as a risk factor for fluconazole-resistant Candida bloodstream infection. Antimicrobial agents and chemotherapy, 56;2518-23.

C.K.S Ong, D. P. (2007). An Evidence-Based Update on Nonsteroidal Anti-Inflammatory Drugs. Clinical Medical Research, 5(1):19-34.

Chang, B. P. (1987). Pharmacology and Applications of Chinese Materia Medica vol 2. World Scientific, 967-974.

Charles W. Saunders, A. S. (2012). Malassezia Fungi Are Specialized to Live on Skin and Associated with Dandruff, Eczema, and other Skin Diseases. PLOS Pathogens, 8(6):e1002701.

Chen, J. (2009). Traditional Chinese Medicine and Infectious Disease. Acupuncture Today, Vol 10, issue 08.

chief), L. D. (2000-06). Chinese Herbal Medicine. Shanghai: Shanghai scientific and technical Publishers.

Collaboration, A. T. (2002). Collaborative meta-analysis of randomised trials of antiplatelet therapy for prevention of death, myocardial infarction, and stroke in high-risk patients. BMJ, 324(7329):71-86.

Dajani EZ, S. T. (2016). Overview of the preclinical pharmacological properties of Nigella sativa (black seeds): a complementary drug with historical and clinical significance. J Physiol Pharmacol, 67(6):801-817.

Das S, D. D. (2007). Anti-inflammatory responses of resveratrol. Inflammatory Allergy Drug Targets, 6(3):168-73.

Diana N. Obanda, D. R. (2016). An extract of Urtica dioica L. mitigates obesity-induced insulin resistance in mice skeletal muscle via protein phosphate 2A(PPSA). Scientific Reports.

Elisya Y, K. L. (2014). Tablet formation of the ethyl acetate soluble extract of soursop (Annona muricata) leaves. Asian J Appl Sci, 2:323-329.

Fal AM, C. F. (2016). Antiviral activity of the "Virus Blocking Factor" (VBF) derived i.a. from Pelargonium extract and Sambucus juice against different human-pathogenic cold viruses in vitro. Wiad Lek, :69(3 pt 2):499-511.

Faridah Hussin, S. A. (2014). The centella asiatica juice effects on DNA damage, apoptosis and gene expression in hepatocellular carcinoma (HCC). BMC Complement Altern Med, 14: 32.

Florence NT, B. M. (2014). Antidiabetic and antioxidant effects of Annona muricata ( Annonaceae), aqueous extract on streptozotocin induced diabetic rats. J of Ethnopharmacol, 151:784-790.

Foster K, Y. N.-W. (2017). Reliance on medicinal plant therapy among cancer patients in Jamaica. Cancer Causes Control, s10552-017-0924-9.

Frøkiær H, H. L. (2012). Astragalus root and elderberry fruit extracts enhance the IFN-β stimulatory effects of Lactobacillus acidophilus in murine-derived dendritic cells. PLoS One, 7(10):e47878.

Fungal Diseases: Candidiasis. (2015, 6 12). Retrieved from Centers for Disease Control and Prevention: www.cdc.gov

Gerd Bendas, L. B. (2012). Cancer Cell Adhesion and Metastasis: Selectins, Integrins, and the Inhibitory Potential of Heparins. International Journal of Cell Biology, Article ID 676731, 10 pages.

Guo, Z., Liu, X.-M., Zhang, Q.-X., Tin, F.-W., Zhang, H., Zhang, H.-P., & Chen, W. (2012). Effects of Inulin on the Plasma Lipid Profile Of Normolipidemic and Hyperlipidemic subjects. Clinical Lipidology, 7(2):215-222.

Gutierrez, M. A. (1998). Medicinal Use Of The Latin Food Staple Nopales: The Prickly Pear Cactus. Nutrition Bytes.

Hansra DM, S. O. (2014). Patient with metastatic breast cancer achieves stable disease for 5 years on graviola and xeloda after progressing on multiple lines of therapy. Adv. Breast Cancer Res, 3:84-87.

Hiroaki Shime, M. Y. (2008). Tumor-Secreted Lactic Acid Promotes IL-23/IL-17 Proinflammatory Pathway. Journal of Immunology, vol .180 no.11 7175-7183.

Hort W, M. P. (2011). Malassezia Virulence determinants. CURR OPIN INFECT DIS, 24:100-105.

Hsien-Yi Wang, W.-C. K.-J.-H.-H.-J. (2014). Differential anti-diabetic effects and mechanism of action of charantin rich extract of Taiwanese Momordica charantia between type 1 and type 2 diabetic mice. In W.-C. K.-J.-H.-H.-J. Hsien-Yi Wang, Food and Chemical Toxicology (pp. 347-356). Elsevier.

Hsuan SL, C. S. (2009). The cytotoxicity to leukemia cells and antiviral effects of Isatis indigotica extracts on pseudorabies virus. Journal Ethnopharmacology, 123(1):61-7.

Huseini HF, L. B. (2006). The efficacy of Silybum marianum (L) Gaertn. (SILYMARIN) in the treatment of type 2 diabetes: a randomized, double-blind, placebo-controlled, clinical trial. Phytother Res, 20(12):1036-9.

Invasive Candiasis. (2015, 6 12). Retrieved from Centers for Disease Control and Prevention: www.cdc.gov

J, P.-R. E.-O.-N.-M.-C. (2014). The effect of nopal on postprandial blood glucose, incretins, and antioxidant activity in Mexican patients with type 2 diabetes after consumption of 2 different breakfasts. Journal of the Academy of Nutrition and Diabetics.

J. Giri, T. S. (1985). Effect of Jamun Seed extracts on Alloxan-Induced Diabetes in Rats. Journal of the Diabetic Association of India vol 25, 9-14.

Jean-Luc Blond, D. L.-F.-L. (2000). An envelope Glycoprotein of the human endogenous retrovirus HERV-W is expressed in the human Placenta and Fuses Cells expressing the type D mammalian retrovirus receptor. Journal of Virology.

Kamtchouing P, K. S. (2006). Antidiabetic activity of methanol/methylene chloride stem bark extracts of terminalia superba and Canarium schweinfurthii on streptozotocin induced diabetic rats. Journal of Ethnopharmacology, 306-309.

Kashmira J. Gohil, J. A. (2010). Pharmacological Review on Centella asiatica: A Potential Herbal Cure-all. Indian Journal of Pharm Sciences, 72(5): 546–556.

Kassaian N, A. L. (2009, January). effects of fenugreek on blood glucose and lipid profiles in type 2 diabetic patients. US National Library of Medicine National Institutes of Health, 79(1):34-9. doi:10.1024/0300-9831.79.1.34.

Khanh V, D. C.-H. (2015). Gallic Acid regulates body weight and glucose homeostasis through AMPK activation. Endocrinology, Volume 156, issue 1, 157-168.

Khanna, A., Chander, R., & Kapoor, N. a. (1994). Phytother. Res, 403.

Kim DC, K. S. (2012). Anticoagulant activities of curcumin and its derivative. BMB Rep, 45(4):221-6.

Kimmatkar N, T. V. (2003). Efficacy and tolerability of Boswellia serrata extract in the treatment of osteoarthritis of knee- a randomized double-blind placebo controlled trial. Phytomedicine, 10(1):3-7.

Kostas ET, W. D. (2016). Selection of yeast strains for bioethanol production from UK seaweeds. J Appl Phycol, 28:1427-1441.

Kulshreshtha G, B. T. (2016). Red Seaweeds Sarcodiotheca gaudichaudii and Chondrus crispus down Regulate Virulence Factors of Salmonella Enteritidis and Induce Immune Responses in Caenorhabditis elegans. Front Microbio, 7:421.

L, L. (2006). Review article: gastrointestinal bleeding with low dose aspirin, what's the risk? Aliment Pharmacol Ther, 24(6):897-908.

Li Z, L. L. (2017). Radix isatidis Polysaccharides Inhibit Influenza a Virus and Influenza A Virus Induced Inflammation via Suppresion of Host TLR3 Signaling In Vitro. Molecules, 22(1).pii E116.

Lockhart SR, I. N. (2012). Species identification and antifungal susceptibility testing of Candida bloodstream isolates from population-based surveillance studies in two US cities from 2008 to 2011. Journal of clinical microbiology, 50:3435-42.

Lowe HI, F. C. (2014). Specific RSK kinase inhibition by dibenzyl trisulfide and implication for therapeutic treatment of cancer. Anticancer Res, 34(4):1637-41.

M.Markovitz, D. (2014). Reverse Genomics and Human Endogenous Retroviruses. Transactions of the American Clinical and Climatological Association, 125:57-63.

Magee KD, C. S. (2008). Heparin versus placebo for acute coronary syndromes. Cochrane Database Syst Rev, 2:CD003462.

Maneewan C, M. A. (2014). Effects of dietary Centella asiatica (L.) Urban on growth performance, nutrient digestibility, blood composition in piglets vaccinated with Mycoplasma hyopneumoniae. Anim Sci J, 85(5):569-74.

Mann, D. (1997). Antifungal agent lowers PSA levels, study finds. Medical Tribune.

Maria de Fatima Arrigoni-Blank, E. G. (2004). Anti-inflammatory and analgesic activity of Peperomia pellucida (L.) HBK (Piperaceae). Journal of Ethnopharmacology, 215-218.

Mckenna, M. (2017, January 13). After Years of Debate, The FDA finally curtails antibiotic use in livestock. Retrieved from www.newsweek.com

Medications that weaken Your immune system and fungal infections. (2017, 1 25). Retrieved from Centers for Disease Control and Prevention: www.cdc.gov

Mei Zhang, L. C.-M. (2006). Growth-inhibitory effects of a β-glucan from the mycelium of Poria cocos on human breast carcinoma MCF-7 cells: Cell-cycle arrest and apoptosis induction. Oncology Reports, 637-643.

Melody Ryan, G. C. (1999). Preventing stroke in patients with transient ischemic Attacks. American Family Physician, 2329-2336.

Minh Q Ngo, P., D, N. N., & Sachin A Shah, P. D. (2010). Oral Aloe Vera for Treatment of Diabetes Mellitus and Dyslipidemia. American Journal of Health-System Pharmacy, 67(21):1804-1811.

Moghadamtousi SZ, R. E. (2015). The chemopotential effect of Annona muricata leaves against azoxymethane-induced colonic aberrant crypt foci in rats and the apoptotic effect of acetogenin annomuricin E in HT-29 cells. PLoS ONE, 10.1371.

Moore-Landecker. (1996). Fundamentals of Fungi. Benjamin Cummings.

Moreno Franco B, L. L. (2014). Soluble and insoluble dietary fibre intake and risk factors for metabolic syndrome and cardiovascular disease in middle-aged adults. The AWHS cohort, 30(6):1279-88.

Ms. Sejal Patel, D. J. (2016). A review on a miracle fruit of Annona muricata. Journal of Pharmacognosy and Phytochemistry, 5(1):137-148.

N'gouemo P, K. B.-N. (1997). Effects of ethanol extract of induced tissue lipid peroxidation. Phytother. Res, 11:326-327.

Nilesh Amatya, A. V. (2017). IL-17 Signaling: The Yin and the Yang. Trends in Immunology, Volume 38, Issue 5, p310–322.

PR Cheeke, S. P. (2006). Anti-inflammatory and anti-arthritic effects of yucca schidigera: A review. Journal of Inflammation, 3:6.

Prasad S, A. B. (2011). Tumeric, the Golden Spice: From Traditional Medicine to Modern Medicine. Herbal Medicine: Biomolecular and clinical Aspects 2nd edition, chapter 13.

Protobase- pLANT rESOURCES OF tROPICAL aFRICA. (n.d.). Retrieved from http://www.prota.org.

Puri, H. (1999). Neem the Divine Tree, Azadirachta indices. Amsterdam: Harwood Academic Publishers.

Puri, H. (2003). Rasayana: Ayurvedic herbs for longevity and rejuvenation. London and New York: Taylor and Francis.

Purushothaman, K. M. (1985). Biological profile of plumbagin. Bulletin Medico Ethnobotanical Research, 177-188.

Qi-min Zhan1, ,. L.-h.-m.-w.-b. (2012). Recent Advances in Cancer Research and Therapy. Elsevier, 493-534.

R Andrew Moore, S. D. (2006). Tolerability and adverse events in clinical trials of celecoxib in osteoarthritis and rheumatoid arthritis: systematic review and meta-analysis of information from company clinical trial reports. Arthritis Research and Therapy, 8(1):401.

Ramirez-Garcia A, R. A.-U.-D.-d. (2016). Candida albicans and cancer. Can this yeast induce cancer development or progression. Crit Rev Microbiol, 42(2):181-93.

Rani P, K. (2004). Antimicrobial evaluation of some medicinal plants for their anti-enteric potential against multi-drug resistant Salmonella typhi. Phytother Res., 18(8):670-3.

Roopesh Jain, S. K. (2010). Ayurveda and cancer. Pharmacognosy Research, 2(6): 393–394.

Sharma I., G. D. (1991). Hypolipidaemic and antiatherosclerotic effect of plumbagin in rabbits. Indian Journal of Physiology and Pharmacology, 35,10-14.

Shim, H. e. (1998). A unique glucose dependant apoptotic pathway induced by c-Myc. . Proceedings of The National Academy of Science, 95;1511-1516.

Shujie Cheng, I. E. (2013). Triterpenes from Poria cocos suppress growth and invasiveness of pancreatic cancer cells through the downregulation of MMP-7. International Journal of Oncology, 1869-1874.

Siddiqui, M. (2011). Boswellia Serrata, A Potential Antiinflammatory Agent: An Overview. Indian Journal of Pharm Sci, 73(3):255-261.

Stanska R, S. R.-V. (2005). survey of acyclovir-resistant herpes simplex virus in the Netherlands: prevalence and characterization. J Clin Virol, 32(1):7-18.

Subramani R, G. E. (2016). Nimbolide inhibits pancreatic cancer growth and metastasis through ROS-mediated apoptosis and inhibition of epithelial-to-mesenchymal transition. Sci Rep.

Tandon, S., Rastogi, R., Shukla, R., Kapoor, N., & Srimal, R. D. (1995). Med Sci. Res, 23, 515.

Tayyab F, L. S. (2012). A review: Medicinal plants and its impact on Diabetes. World J Pharm Res, 1(4):1019-1046.

Teeguarden, R. (1985). CHINESE TONIC HERBS. Japan Publications.

Tiejun Zhao, Q. S. (2015). Anticancer Properties of Phyllanthus emblica (Indian Gooseberry). Oxid Med Cell Longev, 2015: 950890.

Treatment of Fungal Infections Led to Leukemia Remission. (1999). Medical Tribune.

Types of Fungal Diseases. (2017, 1 25). Retrieved from Center for Disease Control and Prevention: www.cdc.gov

Ung-Kyu Choi, O.-H. L.-W.-L.-C. (2010). Hypolipidemic and Antioxidant Effects of Dandelion(Taraxacum officinale) Root and Leaf on Cholesterol-Fed Rabbits. Int J Mol Sci, 11(1):67-78.

Vallabhaneni S, C. A. (2015). Epidemiology and Risk Factors for Echinocandin Nonsusceptible Candida glabrata Bloodstream Infections: Data from a Large Multisite Population-Based Candidemia Surveillance Program, 2008-2014. Open Forum Infect Diseases, 2(4):ofv163.

Vonshak, B. O.-G. (2003). Screening South Indian medicinal plants for antifungal activity against cutaneous pathogens. Phytother Res., 17(9):1123-5.

Walters Jae, G. P.-B. (2005). Systematic corticosteroids for acute exacerbations of chronic obstructive pulmonary disease. Cochrane Database Syst Rev, 25(1):CD001288.

Wang, Y. (1983). Pharmacology and Applications of Chinese Materia Medica. Beijing: Peoples Health Publisher.

Warburg O, O. Y. (1930). Metabolism of Tumors.

Wu T, G. J. (2017). Asiatic acid inhibits lung cancer cell growth in vitro and in vivo by destroying mitochondria. Acta Pharm Sin B, 7(1):65-72.

Xian YF, M. Q. (2011). Comparison of the anti-inflammatory effect of Cortex Phellodendri Chinensis and Cortex Phellodendri Amurensis in 12-O- tetradecanoyl-phorbol-13-acetate-induced ear edema in mice. Journal of Ethnopharmacology, 137(3):1425-30.

Xing, W. Y. (1642). Wen Yi Lun (Discussion of Warm Disease).

Zhaoxia Liu, L. W. (2013). Hypoglycemic Activity and Antioxidative Stress of Extracts and Corymbiferin from swertia bimaculata in votro and in vivo. Evidence-based complementary and alternative medicine volume 2013, 12 pages.